International Perspectives on Racial and Ethnic Mixedness and Mixing

People from a 'mixed' or 'inter' racial and ethnic background, and people partnering and parenting across different racial and ethnic backgrounds, are of increasing political, public and intellectual interest internationally. Contributors to this interdisciplinary collection interrogate notions of mixedness and mixing, and challenge stereotypical assumptions. They advance debates in the field through illuminating the complexity of specific historical trajectories, administrative practices and lived experience.

Recurrent themes woven throughout the chapters include:

- boundaries and categorisation in terms of administration and government, and also of lived experience;
- the explicit and implicit politics of mixedness and mixing in terms of nation state interests, agendas and policies, as well as 'on-the-ground' social relations;
- the ways that mixedness and mixing shift in meaning and implications across time and place, shaped by different national, regional and/or local contexts.

This volume shows that who is and is not 'mixed' is contested and understandings of mixedness and mixing, however conceived, need to be situated in the larger complex of ideas about race and its classification. *International Perspectives on Racial and Ethnic Mixedness and Mixing* is an invaluable book for students and scholars of race and ethnicity.

Rosalind Edwards is Professor of Sociology at the University of Southampton, UK.

Suki Ali is Senior Lecturer in the Department of Sociology at the London School of Economics, UK.

Chamion Caballero is Senior Research Fellow at London South Bank University, UK.

Miri Song is Professor of Sociology at the University of Kent, UK.

Relationships & Resources
Series Editors: Janet Holland and Rosalind Edwards

A key contemporary political and intellectual issue is the link between the relationships that people have and the resources to which they have access. When people share a sense of identity, hold similar values, trust each other and reciprocally do things for each other, this has an impact on the social, political and economic cohesion of the society in which they live. So, are changes in contemporary society leading to deterioration in the link between relationships and resources, or new and innovative forms of linking, or merely the reproduction of enduring inequalities? Consideration of relationships and resources raises key theoretical and empirical issues around change and continuity over time as well as time use, the consequences of globalisation and individualisation for intimate and broader social relations, and location and space in terms of communities and neighbourhoods. The books in this series are concerned with elaborating these issues and will form a body of work that will contribute to academic and political debate.

Available titles include:

Marginalised Mothers
Exploring working-class experiences of parenting
Val Gillies

Sibling Identity and Relationships
Sisters and brothers
Rosalind Edwards, Lucy Hadfield, Helen Lucey and Melanie Mauthner

Teenagers' Citizenship
Experiences and education
Susie Weller

Researching Families and Communities
Social and generational change
Edited by Rosalind Edwards

Interdependency and Care over the Lifecourse
Sophia Bowlby, Linda McKie, Susan Gregory and Isobel MacPherson

Transnational Families
Ethnicities, identities and social capital
Harry Goulbourne, Tracey Reynolds, John Solomos and Elisabetta Zontini

International Perspectives on Racial and Ethnic Mixedness and Mixing
Edited by Rosalind Edwards, Suki Ali, Chamion Caballero and Miri Song

Forthcoming titles include:

Moving On
The changing lives of young people after parental divorce
Bren Neale and Jennifer Flowerdew

Critical Approaches to Care
Understanding caring relations, identities and cultures
Edited by Chrissie Rogers and Susie Weller

International Perspectives on Racial and Ethnic Mixedness and Mixing

Edited by
Rosalind Edwards, Suki Ali, Chamion Caballero and Miri Song

Routledge
Taylor & Francis Group
LONDON AND NEW YORK

First published 2012
by Routledge
2 Park Square, Milton Park, Abingdon, Oxon, OX14 4RN

Simultaneously published in the USA and Canada by Routledge
711 Third Avenue, New York, NY 10017

Routledge is an imprint of the Taylor & Francis Group, an informa business

British Library Cataloguing in Publication Data
A catalogue record for this book is available from the British Library

Library of Congress Cataloging in Publication Data
International perspectives on racial and ethnic mixedness and mixing / edited by Rosalind Edwards … [et al.].
p. cm. – (Relationships & resources)
Includes bibliographical references.
1. Multiculturalism. 2. Racially mixed people. 3. Race. 4. Ethnic groups.
I. Edwards, Rosalind.
HM1271.I589 2012
305.8 – dc23
2011047145

ISBN: 978-0-415-59804-0 (hbk)
ISBN: 978-0-203-11834-4 (ebk)

Typeset in Times New Roman
by Taylor & Francis Books

MIX
Paper from responsible sources
FSC® C013604
www.fsc.org

Printed and bound in Great Britain by
CPI Group (UK) Ltd, Croydon, CR0 4YY

Contents

Figures

Tables

Contributors

Suki Ali is Senior Lecturer in the Department of Sociology at the London School of Economics. Her research interests include racialisation and embodiment, families, visual culture and racial science. Her current research continues to explore the meanings and experiences of mixedness and mixing using feminist postcolonial theory.

Peter Aspinall is Reader in Population Health, School of Social Policy, Sociology & Social Research, University of Kent, Honorary Special Advisor to the London Health Observatory on ethnicity inequalities, and Research Advisor to the National Institute of Health Research Research Design Service South East. He has pursued an active research interest in ethnicity terminology and classifications over the last 20 years and has published around 60 peer-reviewed journal articles in this and allied fields. Between 1994 and 1999 he was the Office for National Statistics' (ONS) National Convenor for the ethnicity question set in the 2001 Census Development Programme and is currently an Academic Advisory Group Member of the ONS Advisory Group on Language, Ethnicity, Religion, and National Identity for the 2011 Census. He is a Director and Trustee for a mixed-race charity.

Chamion Caballero is Senior Research Fellow at London South Bank University. Her research interests include issues relating to mixed racial and ethnic people, couples and families, as well as ethnic and racial minority issues more generally. Published research in these areas include reports for the former Department for Education and Skills (*Understanding the Educational Needs of Mixed Heritage Pupils* (with Leon Tikly, Jo Haynes and John Hill, 2004)) and the Joseph Rowntree Foundation (*Parenting 'Mixed' Children: Negotiating Difference and Belonging in Mixed Race, Ethinicity and Faith Families* (with Rosalind Edwards and Shuby Puthussery, 2008)). Her research with Peter Aspinall on mixed-race people, families and couples in early twentieth-century Britain is the foundation of the BBC2 television series *Mixed Britannia*.

Rosalind Edwards is Professor of Sociology at the University of Southampton. Her research interests are concerned with family issues and experiences, including 'mixed' family lives, taking a critical and feminist perspective. She has published widely in this field. She is also founding and co-editor of the *International Journal of Social Research Methodology*.

Mark Ellis is Professor of Geography and Director of the Center for Studies in Demography and Ecology at the University of Washington, Seattle. His research investigates questions associated with immigration, internal migration, local labour markets and residential segregation.

Steven R. Holloway is Professor of Geography at the University of Georgia. His research centres on critical race studies, with specific foci on residential segregation, racial mixing and housing market processes. He also studies the contingent nature of racial socialisation and collective efficacy across the urban continuum and has emerging interests in the socio-racial dimensions of the urban–nature nexus.

Ilan Katz is Professor and Director of the Social Policy Research Centre (SPRC) at the University of New South Wales, Sydney. He has directed the SPRC since 2005. After graduating as a social worker in South Africa he started his career as a social worker in the UK. He then worked as a research manager in the NGO and as a civil servant before returning to research full time. He completed his PhD 'The Development of Racial Identity in Children of Mixed Heritage' at Brunel University in 1994. His research interests include evidence-based policy, migration, race and ethnicity, evaluation, prevention, early intervention and family support, parenting, child protection, social inclusion, comparative child welfare systems, children in and out of home care, and disability.

Lisa McKenzie currently holds an Early Years Leverhulme Research Fellowship at the University of Nottingham within the School of Sociology and Social Policy. Her research is a re-study of the 1970 Coates and Silburn St Anns 'Poverty' study, focusing upon the changing shapes of community, family and belonging in contemporary Britain. This is a continuation of a four-year study which was set on the St Anns council estate in Nottingham focusing upon white mothers to mixed-race children, and the inter-relationships between class, race, gender and place. She has been commissioned by Policy Press to write a monograph relating to the research in St Anns, expected publication January 2013.

Minelle Mahtani is Associate Professor in the Department of Geography and Planning, and Program in Journalism, at University of Toronto. She completed her PhD at University College London and is a Fellow of the Royal Canadian Geographical Society. She has finished a manuscript on women of mixed race in Toronto, Canada and has published on multiracial identity in a variety of journals, including *Ethnicities* and *Social Identities*, and is one of the editors of the forthcoming collection, *Global Mixed Race*.

Ann Morning is Associate Professor of Sociology at New York University. Her research interests include race, demography and the sociology of science, especially as they pertain to census classification and to individuals' concepts of racial difference. Her doctoral thesis was a co-recipient of the American Sociological Association's 2005 Dissertation Award, and was published in 2011 by the University of California Press with the title *The Nature of Race: How Scientists Think and Teach about Human Difference.* She was the recipient of a 2008–9 Fulbright research award to visit the University of Milan-Bicocca, and has consulted on racial statistics for the European Commission in Brussels and the US Census Bureau. She holds her PhD in Sociology from Princeton University.

Lucinda Platt is Professor of Sociology and Director of the Millennium Cohort Study at the Institute of Education, University of London. A quantitative socialist with a particular interest in longitudinal analysis, her main research areas are child poverty and ethnic inequalities. She has published extensively in these areas. As well as being PI of the Millennium Cohort Study, a longitudinal study of 19,000 children born in 2000/2001, she leads the ethnicity strand of the major UK household panel study, Understanding Society.

Mateja Sedmak is Senior Research Associate at the Science and Research Centre, University of Primorska, Slovenia and Associate Professor in the Department of Cultural Studies at the Faculty of Humanities at the same university. She obtained her PhD from the University of Ljubljana, Slovenia. Her research interests include ethnic studies, intercultural contacts, minorities issues, sociology of family, sociology of everyday life, and ethnically mixed families. She is the author of *Blood and Culture: Ethnically Mixed Marriages in Slovene Istria* (2002, Založba Annales) and co-author of *Radici e le ali: La vita familiare in Slovenia* (*Root and Wings: Family Life in Slovenia*, 2005, Qualecultura) and several articles. She has edited several volumes, including *Between Public and Private: Women on the Labour Market* (2007, Založba Annales), *Images of Life along the Border* (2009, Založba Annales) and *Discussions on Interculturality* (2010, Založba Annales).

Miri Song is Professor of Sociology at the University of Kent. Her research interests include race and mixed race, racisms, and migration (especially second generation migrants). She is the author of *Choosing Ethnic Identity* (Polity Press) and *Helping Out: Children's Labor in Ethnic Businesses* (Temple University Press). She is currently writing (with Peter Aspinall) a book called *Mixed Race Identities* (forthcoming with Palgrave Macmillan).

Anne Unterreiner graduated from the Political Science Institute of Lyon, and then obtained a Masters degree in Sociology at the School for Advanced Studies in the Social Sciences (EHESS), Paris, France, where she currently is reading for a PhD. She is affiliated to the Research Team on Social Inequality (ERIS), Maurice Halbwachs Center (CMH), Paris, France, with Serge Paugam as her advisor. Her main focus is on mixedness. Her graduation thesis in the Political Science Institute of Lyon was entitled 'The Family Background, Education and Identity of French-Japanese Children in Japan'; her Masters thesis was about 'The Identity of Bi-National Couples' Children in France'; and now, as a PhD student, she is focusing on 'The Integration and Identity of Mixed People: A Comparative Study in Europe'. She is using both quantitative and qualitative data studying mixedness in a comparative research.

Richard Wright holds the Orvil E. Dryfoos Chair in Public Affairs and is Professor of Geography at Dartmouth College, USA. His research and teaching primarily concerns racial mixing in households and neighbourhoods, regional labour market processes, nativism and the racialisation of immigrants (and the native born).

1 Introduction

Approaches to racial and ethnic mixedness and mixing

Rosalind Edwards, Miri Song, Chamion Caballero and Suki Ali

People from a 'mixed' or 'inter' racial and ethnic background, and people partnering and parenting across different racial and ethnic backgrounds – the mixedness and mixing of the title of this book – are of increasing political, public and intellectual interest internationally. In many countries discussion often focuses on assertions about identity (and the rights associated), black/white mixes and pathologically focused research agenda. The different racial histories of the countries concerned inform how these debates are understood and played out. Nonetheless, across contexts, mixedness and mixing often are significant in the light of debates about multi-culturalism, and 'race' and ethnicity more broadly, albeit in quite different ways.

The contributors to this volume discuss these debates and literatures as these relate to the aspects of mixedness and mixing that they address, so we do not provide a comprehensive background review of the burgeoning work in the broad field in this Introduction. For now, we note that, on the one hand, images of racial, ethnic and faith diversity are posed in opposition to societal unity and solidarity, with assertions that these differences create a crisis of cohesive national social trust (e.g. Goodhart 2004; Putnam 2007). On the other hand, there are arguments that such sweeping portrayals of segregation and conflict ignore the reality of ongoing local interactions between a mix of minority and majority racial, ethnic and religious cultures, where multi-culture is an ordinary, unremarkable, feature of everyday social life (Gilroy 2004; Hall 2000).

Mixing and mixedness are often posed as fraught with difficulty in terms of personal relationships and psychologies. The notion of 'culture clash' is used frequently to explain the supposedly transient and problematic nature of mixed relationships, and parents of mixed-race and ethnic children generally are subject to enduring negative assumptions regarding their backgrounds, relationships and parenting skills (see reviews in Caballero *et al.* 2008, and Crippen and Brew 2007). People from mixed backgrounds themselves have been viewed in oppositional ways (see review in Caballero 2005). On the one hand, they have been regarded as genetically weak and culturally confused – consigned to a marginal and tragic 'between two worlds' status. Disproportionate numbers of mixed children in fostering and adoptive care, or at risk of educational underachievement, are often associated with 'identity confusion'. On the other hand, there are arguments that mixed people have a stronger genetic profile, are more beautiful, healthy and intelligent. These sub-normal and supra-normal conceptualisations each stem from the same premise that people from mixed backgrounds are somehow different to 'mono-racial' people.

The legacy of conceptions of people from mixed-race backgrounds as 'confused' and liable to identity crisis has influenced much research on the topic. In the UK and USA, for example, some work has engaged with the question of whether or not, in particular, white parents (especially white lone mothers) have the ability to raise their mixed black–white children with a 'healthy' sense of self (see reviews in Caballero 2010; Harman 2010; Twine 2010). One strand of this literature, which has been very influential on adoption and fostering practice, can be characterised as 'pro-race' (Caballero 2005). A 'pro-race' position tends to understand mixedness in dualistic black–white terms, and contends that people of black and white parentage should understand themselves as, and be raised as, black, since it is presumed that this is inevitably how they will be perceived by society (e.g. Banks 1996; Prevatt-Goldstein 1999). Another strand, still working within a 'pro-race' approach but challenging this view, argues that mixed-race people need to be raised to recognise both or all of their heritages for a healthy identity (e.g. Milan and Keiley 2000; Oriti *et al.* 1996). Alternative and emerging perspectives, which have had less influence on policy and practice, take more of a 'post-race' approach. They stress that other social identifiers, such as gender, class and nationhood, are just as important as race in creating a sense of self for mixed people. This often is integrally linked with arguments that mixedness is a means to deconstruct racial categorisation, and that the contextual specifics and fluidity of a mixed identity needs to be acknowledged (for example, Ali 2003; Olumide 2002; Song 2003).

While attention to mixedness and mixing is growing rapidly internationally and across disciplines, however, some debates in the field have become somewhat preoccupied with prescriptive assertions about identity; black–white mixes; and pathologically focused research agenda. This is holding back the development of theoretical perspectives and intellectually shaped empirical evidence that can deal with complexity and normalcy, and of cross-disciplinary exchanges and learning. In this context, as researchers whose work addresses various aspects of mixedness and mixing, we wanted to go beyond these preoccupations and parameters. We sought to build on previous collections that have de-problematised mixedness and mixing (including Parker and Song 2001; Root 1996; Williams-Léon and Nakashima 2001; Winters and DeBose 2003), and continue the challenge to stereotypical assumptions through illuminating the complexity of historical trajectories, administrative practices and lived experience. In particular, we wanted to make links across disciplines and learn from nuances of issues about mixedness and mixing across time and place. The result is an edited collection that brings together internationally well-respected researchers addressing mixedness and mixing who work in different disciplinary fields.

The contributors to this volume draw on a variety of disciplinary approaches. From a sociological perspective, for example, authors explore administrative categorisations of mixedness or lack of them in various national contexts, shifting political and experiential boundaries around identity, and intersections of race and class; from a demographic perspective they examine the variables collected about mixed people, and the social-economic characteristics of those who choose to identify as mixed; and from a geographical perspective they look at the way that the racial composition of neighbourhoods plays into assessment of and options for mixed identities. Bringing together sociological, political and historical perspectives, our contributors also consider the history of mixedness and mixing in specific contexts, and the way that this is shot through with the particular national and regional politics of race relations. For some, such multi- or inter-disciplinarity is captured in ideas about 'Mixed-Race Studies', or a comprehensive 'Critical Mixed-Race Theory'. Others work within their primary discipline, pursuing for example sociologies of race and/or family, geographies of race and/or urban geographies. And some raise knotty issues around the use and implications of a transcendent and coherent mixed-race identity in disciplinary, political or experiential terms.

Within the context of this vibrant collection of disciplinary fields, the edited collection is important in the breadth and depth of its spatial coverage. At the level of breadth, this ranges across global comparisons of regions' and nation states' classifications of mixed people; to particular national comparisons such as between Australia and the UK to pull out the dimensions of difference shaping understandings of mixedness in two socially and culturally similar societies, or between understandings of the nation, the others and mixedness in Germany, France and Britain; as well as specific national foci on, for example, Britain, Canada, Slovenia and the USA. At the level of depth, there are intensive explorations of regions and neighbourhoods.

The collection provides both new understandings of familiar material through different perspectives as well as covering new ground. A key feature of the volume is that while there are different sorts of consideration of the continuing implications of black and white mixing and mixedness – such as shifts over time in racial classification and (lack of) recognition of mixedness, or the relationship between race, class and social value – the contributions move beyond the black/white binary to encompass and address other forms of racial and ethnic mixing. Notably there is attention to within-race mixing across ethnic difference.

Also of interest is the range of methods adopted by our contributing authors: quantitative and qualitative, secondary and primary. The chapters variously draw on analysis of secondary material that runs from extensive large-scale quantitative data sets to intensive archived visual and written materials, or on analysis of primary survey and/or in-depth interview data.

Methodological issues are considered as a topic in themselves. Contributors consider the ways that researchers both create and reinforce particular versions of mixedness in and through different national large-scale datasets, and also the intersection of identity boundaries and hidden power relations in in-depth interviews with individuals.

As a collection, we hope that this distinctive variety of contributions with a common concern will aid in illuminating the different contexts and concepts underpinning discussions about mixedness and mixing, and play a leading part in taking forward ways of thinking about them. A recurrent theme woven throughout the chapters is that of boundaries and categorisation in terms of administration and government, and also of lived experience. Interlocked with this there are issues, both explicit and implicit, around politics with a capital P in terms of nation state interests, agenda and policies, as well as the lower-case politics of 'on-the-ground' power relations. Another linked and recurring strand relates to the way that mixedness and mixing shift in meaning and implications across time and place. Within one location the boundaries and politics of mixedness and mixing can demonstrate change historically, and categorisations and power relations are not universal but shaped by their different national, regional and/or local contexts.

We begin the collection with an international overview of administrative classifications; an analysis that is shot through with politics and place. Ann Morning identifies and compares the strategies that different national governments take to the classification of mixed people in censuses around the globe. She reviews the terminologies used around race, nationality and so on, and the approaches to the enumeration of mixed people along a continuum from non-recognition, through various forms of category and combinations, to unrestrained recognition. Nations usually channel expressions of mixed identity into a few predetermined census classifications. The result in each case is similar: a particularistic count of those who are willing and able to identify themselves within the parameters of the mixedness categories offered to them, and the exclusion of others. Morning's thematic analysis draws out the way that, while notions of mixedness are widespread across the world, recognition of mixedness everywhere is linked fundamentally to broader and deeper beliefs about racial difference. How mixedness can be identified and categorised is formed by the specific concepts of group difference and state interests that are embedded in the broader systems of cultural meaning and social structure pertaining at the time.

Time and place are also key features of subsequent chapter discussions. Ilan Katz provides a detailed illustration of Morning's argument, in his exploration of how racial mixedness is bounded in and reflective of specific social, cultural and political developments in time and place and part of wider discourses about race. Katz looks at how social, geographical and political context bear on the possibilities for and implications of mixed identities through a contrasting of Australia with the UK – countries that are often presented as socially, politically and culturally similar. However, Katz shows how the specific history of Australian colonisation and migration shapes the racial and ethnic identity options available to people. In particular, he traces the timeline of Australian racial politics and policy as this interacts with 'identity boundaries'. Katz explains how contemporary definition as 'Aboriginal' is grounded not only in self-identification but also acceptance as such by the Indigenous community. The self-collective identification coupling is a response to the anomalies of the previous imposed colour-based classification of first nations. As Katz points out, both the prior centering of race and the current deliberate exclusion of race from the official lexicon have the same implication – a cutting out of acknowledgement and assertions of a mixed identity, in contrast to the official incorporation of mixedness in the UK.

Chamion Caballero examines the intersection between public condemnatory pronouncements of mixing and mixedness and everyday accounts of mixed people and families in Britain between the 1920s and 1950s – a time when fears of 'miscegenation' and the growth of a 'half-caste' population were rife, alongside and as part of general concerns about 'the colour problem'. While Britain may not have introduced anti-miscegenation laws, more informal pressures of social disapproval and segregation were brought to bear to maintain racial boundaries. Yet, as Caballero points out and illustrates, even within this context, mixed couples and their children lived 'ordinary' family and community lives. She argues that looking at archived accounts of personal lives and photographs of families and communities reveals a complex picture of mixing and mixedness in past times, and enables the thread of ordinariness to be drawn through into present time.

Caballero has people partnering and parenting across different racial and ethnic backgrounds as one of her central concerns. The following two chapter contributions also address mixing as well as mixedness, here moving beyond the broad national perspective across time, into the detail of particular contemporary regional and neighbourhood politics and relations. Mateja Sedmak's chapter provides a graphic illustration of the way that place is not static, with the shifting politics of nation state boundaries shaping identity options. Ethnic difference was downplayed in former Yugoslavia in favour of an ideology of equality and co-existence, but with Slovenian independence came a change of nation state boundaries that brought about a change of ethnic boundaries. Families consisting of Slovenes and members of other states of the former Yugoslavia suddenly became ethnically mixed 'international' families living in a xenophobic, nationalistic environment. In a case study of the ethnically plural Istrian region of Slovenia Sedmak reveals how long-standing migrants from areas outside the former Yugoslavia, notably Italy, are accepted in ways that those from former Yugoslavia are not. She shows the implications for life in mixed families from the perspective of both parents and children, for relations within couples, identity options for children, and the attitudes of extended family.

The following two chapters drill down even further into place. Steven R. Holloway, Richard Wright and Mark Ellis examine constructions of race and mixedness at the local level of families in metropolitan neighbourhoods in the US, through an exploration of white–black and white–Asian couples who classify their children as mixed (marking multiple racial categories) in the census. They begin from an ecological framework that sees racial formations and claims to mixedness as shaped simultaneously at the levels of body, family and neighbourhood, to demonstrate that there is a systematic relationship between parents' census category choices for their children and the nature of their neighbourhood. The more diversity and mixing there is in a neighbourhood, the more likely parents in mixed couples are to report their children as multi-racial. Whether or not this relationship between identification and neighbourhood context poses a challenge to the demarcation of racial hierarchy and racial stratification in the US, as they point out, is another matter.

Lisa McKenzie takes us into a British inner city public housing estate for an alternative perspective on the relationship between race, class and social status through a focus on white mothers of mixed-race children living in the St Anns neighbourhood of Nottingham. The world outside the boundaries of St Anns regards its residents as a pathological 'underclass', but inside the estate that the mothers are part of they help create a status and value for themselves and their children through local networks and shared cultural understandings. These sources of value, or cultural capital, are formed around a combination of 'blackness' and 'working-classness'. In contrast, white working-classness is viewed as cultureless and valueless both inside and outside St Anns. Thus in this neighbourhood enclave, an alternative value system exists for white working-class mothers that has mixing and mixedness at its heart – presenting a more complex picture that is part of the contemporary thread of 'ordinariness' signalled by Caballero's historical analysis in her chapter.

The subsequent two chapters move discussion more deeply into aspects of young people's self-identification of mixedness. Lucinda Platt examines the key demographics and characteristics of the British self-identified mixed population to consider both claims of a 'post-race' era of declining ethnic stratification and a distinct 'mixed' experience. She details a comparatively youthful mixed ethnic population who have similar achievements educationally to the majority population but exhibit differences within the mixed group in ways that map onto the minority element of their backgrounds, along with rates of unemployment and studentship that are higher than the majority but again parallel the relevant non-mixed minority. Mixed people are less likely to marry than all other ethnic groups, however – a topic that needs further investigation. As Platt asks, is this an indictor of a modern, forward-looking population, or indicative of enduring social constraints that limit opportunities for partnership? Overall then, this demographic picture of Britain's mixed population indicates neither a lessening of ethnic stratification nor, for the most part, a particular, categorical mixed-group experience.

Miri Song and Peter Aspinall take us further into the experiences of young mixed-race Britons with their exploration of identity boundaries. They examine whether mixed-race young people believe that their chosen identifications are validated by others, and how they respond to others' racial perceptions of them. While a racial mismatch between expressed and observed identifications was a common experience for these individuals, they varied considerably in terms of how they responded to such occurrences. Song and Aspinall carefully detail how young people could feel affronted, enjoy the curiosity or express indifference to the mismatch – with many feeling a sense of belonging inside the national boundary of Britishness. Whether miscategorisation had negative meanings or implications varied according to the group membership assigned, with feelings of injustice and/or annoyance most often expressed by black/white young people who regarded themselves as mixed but who were frequently pigeonholed as black. This is an indication, Song and Aspinall suggest, that the hierarchical boundary between black and white Britons is still entrenched, albeit in flux.

Many of the foregoing contributors to this volume reflect on some of the methodological issues involved in their studies, but the next two contributions to our collection have this as a central concern. They consider aspects of the politics of methodology, secondary and primary respectively. Anne Unterreiner makes the point that extensive knowledge about mixed people depends on time and place in terms of how a society historically and politically understands the boundary crossings involved in mixedness. It is within this context that certain variables are collected that allow the identification of mixed people and are made available to researchers. Unterreiner takes the examples of German, French and British datasets, in each case reviewing how particularistic national histories and conceptions of the markers of 'Us' (the nation) and 'Them' shape the main population surveys. She shows how these particularities present commensurability difficulties for researchers who wish to use large-scale survey datasets in order to make international comparisons of mixed people's characteristics and circumstances. And, as she points out, just as much as national conceptions, policies and political and academic debates shape the nature of the datasets available to secondary researchers, in a circular fashion their categories and analyses of mixed people turn back and shape the social reality of mixedness.

The implications of undertaking open-ended interviews in mixed-race studies where the researcher herself is an 'insider' is explored by Minelle Mahtani, through a critical reflection on her own research process and racialised subject position. She details the shared complicities, rapport and expectations of mutual recognition around mixedness but also around other identities such as gender, class and profession. Mahtani challenges any simplistic notion of insider/outsider identity boundaries and wonders about the implications of an understanding of mixedness that is built on individual mixed-race researchers' access to more 'authentic' experience in in-depth interviews with individual mixed-race people. She explains her discomfort with the fact that this may leave aside unequal power differentials between racialised groups and the way that these shape and are shaped by a mixed-race identity.

Suki Ali engages such discomfort with a reflection upon similar themes of recognition and representation in the final contribution to the volume. Referencing her arguments through the situated contexts of the UK and USA – but raising wider issues – Ali asks challenging questions about the form, purpose and purchase of a mixed-race politics that champions a universalised mixed-race identity; the meaning of community; and rights to self-representation. She argues, as other contributions to this collection attest, that mixed-race identities and experiences are very diverse and interlock with other kinds of social differentiation. They also inherently engage with racialised ideas about given, definable and bounded races and ethnicities, against which a categorical mixed race often is either pathologised or glorified. Thus Ali calls for a politics of mixedness that is situated in and contingent upon recognition of the specifics of societies' racialised hierarchies, and the ways in which these are bound up with other issues of social difference and inequality.

Overall then, across all the contributions to our edited collection, it is clear that understandings of mixedness and mixing – whether these are created through administrative national/racial/ethnic identity categories and political boundaries, or as part of complex everyday local social relations and subtle lived experiences of insider and outsider identity options – need to be situated in the larger complex of ideas about race and its classification. Thus mixedness and mixing will have an important role in the continuing significance (or not) of broader ideas about 'race' and ethnicity. As the contributions to this volume demonstrate, who is and is not 'mixed' is contested. In future, states, researchers and mixed people themselves will need increasingly to question the positioning and experiences of mixed people in highly specific, contextualised ways – rather than assuming that they are some intermediate category perched between so-called mono-racial groups. As 'mixing' continues apace, the entire rationale and means of classifying 'difference' will come under further scrutiny.

References

Ali, S. (2003) *Mixed-Race, Post-Race: Gender, New Ethnicities and Cultural Practices*, Oxford: Berg.

Banks, N. (1996) 'Young single white mothers with black children in therapy', *Clinical Child Psychology and Psychiatry* 1(1): 19–28.

Caballero, C. (2005) "'Mixed race projects': perceptions, constructions and implications of mixed race in the UK and USA", unpublished PhD thesis, University of Bristol.

——(2010) *Lone Mothers of Children from Mixed Racial and Ethnic Backgrounds: A Case Study*, Bristol: SPAN: http://www.spanuk.org.uk/uploads/Microsoft%20Word%20-%20Lone%20Mothers%20of%20Mixed%20Racial%20and%20Ethnic%20Children%20-%20FINAL.pdf [accessed 07.10.11].

Caballero, C., Edwards, R. and Puthussery, S. (2008) *Parenting 'Mixed' Children: Negotiating Difference and Belonging in Mixed Race, Ethnicity and Faith Families*, York: Joseph Rowntree Foundation.

Crippen, C. and Brew, L. (2007) 'Intercultural parenting and the transcultural family: a literature review', *The Family Journal* 15(2): 107–15.

Gilroy, P. (2004) *After Empire: Melancholia or Convivial Culture?* London: Routledge.

Goodhart, D. (2004) 'Too diverse?', *Prospect*, February: http://www.prospect-magazine.co.uk [accessed 30.4.04].

Hall, S. (2000) 'The multi-cultural question', in B. Hesse (ed.) *Unsettled Multiculturalisms*, London: Zed Press.

Harman, V. (2010) 'Social work practice and lone white mothers of mixed parentage children', *British Journal of Social Work* 40(2): 391–406.

Milan, S. and Keiley, M. (2000) 'Biracial youth and families in therapy: issues and interventions', *Journal of Marital and Family Therapy* 26(3): 305–15.

Olumide, J. (2002) *Raiding the Gene Pool: The Social Construction of Mixed Race*, London: Pluto.

Oriti, B., Bibb, A. and Mahboubi, J. (1996) 'Family centred practice with racially/ethnically mixed families', *Families in Society* 77(9): 573–82.

Parker, D. and Song, M. (eds) (2001) *Rethinking 'Mixed Race'*, London: Pluto Press.

Prevatt-Goldstein, B. (1999) 'Direct work with black children with one white parent', in R. Barn (ed.) *Working with Black Children and Adolescents in Need*, London: BAAF.

Putnam, R.D. (2007) '*E Pluribus Unum*: Diversity and community in the twenty-first century', *Scandinavian Political Studies* 30(2): 137–74.

Root, M. (ed.) (1996) *The Multiracial Experience: Racial Borders as the New Frontier*, Thousand Oaks, CA: Sage.

Song, M. (2003) *Choosing Ethnic Identity*, Cambridge: Polity Press.

Twine, F.W. (2010) *A White Side of Black Britain*, Durham, NC: Duke University Press.

Williams-Léon, T. and Nakashima, C. (eds) (2001) *The Sum of Our Parts: Mixed Heritage Asian Americans*, Philadelphia, PA: Temple University Press.

Winters, L. and DeBose, H. (eds) (2003) *New Faces in a Changing America: Multiracial Identity in the 21st Century*, Thousand Oaks, CA: Sage.

2 Multiraciality and census classification in global perspective

Ann Morning[1]

What Maria Root (1996) called "the multiracial experience" has rarely been studied from a comparative perspective. Although scholars of race and ethnicity have long recognized the importance of placing diverse national contexts side by side in order to glean insights about both their similarities and their particularities, mixed-race people have too often slipped through the cracks. To be sure, international comparison has often dwelled on the tendencies of some countries and not others to recognize racial mixture in their populations; notable examples include Nobles (2000) on Brazil and the United States, and Marx (1998) on the same nations as well as South Africa. But in these works, multiracial people are of interest as components of larger systems of racial structure and ideology; it is not their experience in particular that is at the heart of comparative inquiry.

Why this failure to consider multiraciality as a social identity that transcends state borders? I suggest three reasons. First is simply that "mixed-race studies" in general are fairly new as a subfield of social scientific research. Although multiracial people are hardly new as topics of scientific inquiry (Park's "marginal man," for example, dates back to 1928), a solid body of research that focuses on them is a recent phenomenon (Lee and Bean 2004; Thompson 2006). Second, most investigations of multiracial people's identity or classification explore how they are forged by local or national contexts and institutions (see for example Brunsma 2006; DaCosta 2007; Gross 2007; Saada 2002). In other words, such studies have privileged close examination of specific cultures in order to trace the development of local notions of "who" or "what" racially mixed people are. Such findings, however, are rarely juxtaposed with similar observations from many different cultural settings. Finally—and in a related vein—I would argue that scholars have envisioned multiracial people as forming a series of small, unconnected, nation-specific communities—such as Métis in Canada or Eurasians in Vietnam—rather than as a transnational community whose members share the socially meaningful experience of being considered racially mixed. Perhaps a diasporic model that conceives of far-flung groups as being part of a larger whole—such as Indian-origin communities in Africa, Asia, Europe, North America, the Caribbean, and the Pacific—would be a useful model for understanding multiraciality in global perspective.

But perhaps not. The bottom line is that scholars have not seriously asked, in an empirical manner, what we might gain from international exploration of the multiracial experience. As a result, it is hard to say whether a transnational model of multiraciality—which might presume for example a widespread consciousness of being members of a global population—has any utility at present. Regardless of the answer to this question, however, cross-national comparative research would nonetheless benefit current scholarship on mixed-race people for at least two reasons. First, it would entail exposure to diverse systems of racial ideology that would help us better identify the meaningful characteristics of any single one in particular. Second, it would help us analyze the causes and consequences of different approaches to conceptualizing mixed identity.

In this chapter, I take a comparative look at the classification of multiethnic people worldwide by studying how they were enumerated on nearly 140 censuses over the 1995–2004 period. As I explain below, I will use the word *ethnic* as an umbrella term to capture the wide range of descent-related concepts that censuses use, including *race*, *tribe*, *ancestry*, and others. Multiraciality then is just one form of multiethnicity (or "mixedness") that censuses measure. My aim is to identify the strategies that national governments take with respect to mixed people, and investigate how these strategies vary by world region. In short, this project contributes to a map of what might be called "the geography of mixedness." Finally, I draw on this mapping to demonstrate how understandings of multiraciality are shaped—indeed constrained—by local (or national) concepts of race.

Studying census classification worldwide

Why use censuses as a window onto how mixed people are understood and classified around the world? After all, state classification schemes are not the same as everyday folk categories. In the United States, for example, official terminology like "non-Hispanic whites" or the "Asian alone or in combination population" are probably not used very often outside the halls of the Census Bureau. Yet official classification systems do reflect—and shape—those everyday discussions. More importantly for the purposes of this chapter, they offer a clear measure with which to make comparisons across a large number of countries at once.

The research described below is based on a collection of 138 national census questionnaires that were fielded from 1995 to 2004—that is, during the period demographers call "the 2000 census round." Readers who would like greater detail about the data, methodology, and results of this study are encouraged to consult Morning (2008). Nonetheless, a key observation about these data is in order here: as large as this sample is, it covers only 69 percent of the nation states that fielded a census from the mid-1990s to the mid-2000s.

Moreover, this coverage is geographically biased. Europe is best represented, with 100 percent of its censuses included, and Asia (which includes the Middle East), Oceania, and South America are all well-covered, with 79 to 80 percent of the 2000-round censuses of each region included.[2] In contrast, only 51 percent of the censuses fielded in North America (including Central America and the Caribbean) and 42 percent of those conducted in Africa during the 2000 round were located for this sample. As a result, African, Central American, and Caribbean countries' experience with multiethnic enumeration is not adequately reflected below. This is worth keeping in mind since the Caribbean in particular may be a region where censuses acknowledge racial mixture more frequently than elsewhere.

Until this point, I have referred to the experience of multiraciality. However, the term *race* is so often confounded with *ethnicity* (in scholarly, political, media, and everyday discourse) that when studying census enumeration, I cast a wide net and look at questions about "ethnicity," "race," "nationality" (when clearly distinguished from citizenship), "indigenous group" or "tribe," "ancestry"/"descent"/"origin," "cultural group," "community"/"population," "caste," and "colour" or "phenotype." In short, I aim to analyze census classification of groups that are understood to be "communities of descent" (Hollinger 1998), and I use the term *ethnicity* as an umbrella label to include these varied formulations of the basic notion of a descent-based community. Indeed, Weber's (1978: 389) definition of "ethnic groups" conveys a sense of the variety of conceptual forms these may take:

> We shall call "ethnic groups" those human groups that entertain a subjective belief in their common descent because of similarities of physical type or of customs or of both, or because of memories of colonization and migration; this belief must be important for the propagation of group formation; conversely, it does not matter whether or not an objective blood relationship exists.

In other words, some ethnic identities may place greater weight on similarity of physical type (which is central to the race concept) or customs (e.g. "cultural group") or descent (e.g. "ancestry"). The importance accorded to appearance or traditions or historical memories may lead to different conceptions of shared descent. But whether "caste" or "tribe" or "race" is in play, they are all instances of a broader phenomenon of meaning-making around common descent, and it is that range of notions of communities that I sought to investigate on national censuses, and that I refer to using the term *ethnicity* for shorthand.

This means that the study I conducted was really one of multiethnic rather than strictly multiracial census enumeration. Or rather, it is an exploration of the official recognition of "mixedness" regardless of the terms in which groups are locally conceived (for example, as castes, or tribes, or races). Yet the overarching theme of this chapter is multiraciality, that is, mixedness in its specifically racial framing. Because race has a specific set of connotations, multiraciality also carries its own associations, distinct from being multiethnic or multicultural or multinational. Race hinges above all on beliefs about essential biological characteristics (Winant 2001) and thus has specific implications for understandings of multiraciality—ideas, as we will see below, of how individuals acquire their racial characteristics and identities. Hence I distinguish multiraciality from the broader range of types of multiethnicity as a particular theoretical concept. However, when referring to the analysis of censuses I will use the terms *multiethnic* or simply *mixed* people to denote the wide array of labels that official questionnaires employ.

One last comment on the data analyzed below. I did not approach the census questionnaires with a preconceived list of qualifying terms; instead, I worked inductively to include within the project's scope any question that referred to subdivisions in a national population that implied group cohesiveness born of shared ancestry. I did decide from the outset, however, to exclude question items on language, religion, and legal citizenship. Although these could certainly be considered reflections of ethnic affiliation, I judge them to be relatively indirect references to ancestry. (Consider for example how poor an indicator of ethnicity "Native English Speaker" status would be in a multicultural society like the United States.) As a result, the treatment of census enumeration below is based on a particular approach to defining "ethnic" classification, one that yields different results than would a study that incorporated census items on language or religion.

How do censuses count by ethnicity?

Using the method described above, I determined that of the 138 national census questionnaires analyzed, 87 countries or 63 percent employed some form of ethnic classification. (Again, see Morning 2008 for a more detailed discussion of findings.) North America (including Central America and the Caribbean), South America, and Oceania were the regions with the greatest propensity to include ethnicity on their censuses; 82 to 84 percent of the 2000-round censuses fielded in each of those regions counted their populations by ethnicity. While Asia's tendency to enumerate by ethnicity was close to the sample average, both Europe and Africa were much less likely to do so; in both regions, 44 percent of census questionnaires included ethnicity items. As I have suggested in Morning (2008), this relatively low rate of ethnic enumeration may stem from government concerns that such categorization would be detrimental to projects of national unity (and see Rallu, Piché and Simon 2004 for a series of hypotheses regarding country approaches to ethnic classification).

Regions varied too in the terminology used on their census questionnaires, depending on their histories of colonialism, slavery, migration, and political boundary shifts. Overall, references to "ethnicity," "nationality" (as distinct from legal citizenship), "indigenous" status, and "race" predominated; together, these four terms accounted for 90 percent of the descent items on the censuses sampled. The modal term of ethnicity was most frequent in Oceania, where it appeared on 81 percent of the censuses sampled, and least prevalent in South America, where it appeared on only 33 percent.

In contrast, references to "indigenous status" or "tribe" reached their peak in South America (appearing on 67 percent of censuses there), but were absent on European and Asian censuses. Thus indigeneity seemed particularly salient in societies where European colonialism resulted either in considerable *mestizaje* that became the norm against which the indigenous were marked (as in Latin America), or in a European-dominated population in which indigenous people were equally marginalized (e.g. the United States, Canada, Australia, and New Zealand).

Conversely, "nationality" appeared on none of the American censuses (South or North), but figured on more than half of the European censuses. This was particularly true of Eastern Europe, where historical and often war-related movements of political borders and peoples have frequently left groups with allegiances to past or neighbouring governments situated in new or different states (Eberhardt 2003). Moreover, the former Soviet Union's practice of identifying distinct nationalities within its borders extended the equation of nationality with ethnic membership that is still seen in post-USSR states such as Tajikistan, Turkmenistan, and Uzbekistan (Blum and Gousseff 1996).

Finally, "race" is not found on European or Asian censuses, but appears on almost half of those used in North/Central America and the Caribbean. In fact, race as a census item is used virtually exclusively by either New World former slave societies (United States, Anguilla, Bermuda, Brazil, Jamaica, Saint Lucia) and/or their territories (United States Virgin Islands, Puerto Rico, American Samoa, Guam, Northern Mariana Islands). This marked geographic concentration of race terminology may be another reason that multiraciality has not often been researched from an international perspective. The term *race* seems to have less purchase outside the Americas, and thus less immediate salience as the basis for a wide-ranging cross-national comparison.

Census questionnaires also varied notably in the response formats they provided for ethnicity questions. These formats were fairly evenly divided across three types:

1 closed-ended responses (e.g. category checkboxes or code lists);
2 closed-ended with open-ended "Other" option (i.e. permitting the respondent to write in a group name that is not included on the list presented);
3 open-ended (i.e. write-in blanks).

The ways in which respondents are permitted to report their ethnic affiliation is of central importance to the question of how censuses recognize and record mixedness. As the typology above suggests, different response formats offer respondents different amounts of latitude as well as different frameworks for reporting a mixed identity.

Counting mixed people

Among the census questionnaires I studied, five approaches to enumerating mixed people emerged:

1 *Non-recognition.* On some censuses with a closed response set (e.g. checkboxes), registering a mixed identity was simply not an option. This was a rare occurrence, occurring on only six questionnaires (Zambia, Cyprus, Hungary, Costa Rica, Mexico, and New Caledonia). For example, the Mexican census *pertenencia etnica* question asked only whether the respondent belonged to an indigenous group, offering simply "yes / no" response options. In such a framework, registering a multiethnic identity is not possible.

2 *Combination of predetermined categories.* Other censuses with a closed response set permitted individuals to combine predetermined ethnic options. For example, New Zealand's census asked, "Which ethnic group do you belong to? Mark the space *or spaces* which apply to you" (emphasis added). Canada and the United States used the same approach. In these cases, the number and kinds of mixed identities that one can report are limited by the menu of ethnic categories that is offered from which to select. I discuss these limits further below.

3 *"Mixed" category.* Still other censuses with a closed response set included a generic "mixed" category among their options. Examples include the "mixed" category on the censuses of Zimbabwe, Trinidad and Tobago, and Jamaica, and the "*mestizo*" option in Belize and Peru.

4 *Predetermined combinations.* Yet other closed-response census items included among their checkboxes categories that specified particular group combinations (or groups whose label denoted a specific combination). For example, Bermuda's census included "Black and White" and "Black and Other"; the Cook Islands specified "Part Cook Island Maori" as a response option; Singapore included "Eurasian" as a response, and Sri Lanka's census enumerated "Burghers."

5 *Unconstrained recognition.* In contrast to censuses which used closed-ended response formats to enumerate ethnicity, questionnaires that permitted open-ended (i.e. write-in) responses offered total latitude in indicating a mixed identity. These censuses provide the bulk of the opportunity for individuals to report mixed affiliations. Examples of this open-ended approach can be found on the censuses of Mauritius, Senegal, Armenia, China, Iraq, Vietnam, and Russia.[3]

To determine which of these five strategies were most common, and in which regions, I looked at the subset of countries that did not use code lists, because

Table 2.1 Multiple identity classification by region

Census approach to enumerating mixed individuals:	*South America*	*North America*	*Oceania*	*Africa*	*Europe*	*Asia*	*TOTAL*	
	%	%	%	%	%	%	%	*N*
No Recognition	0	17	6	17	6	5	8	*6*
Open-Ended	20	8	31	33	81	84	51	*38*
Allow Mixed Identification	80	75	63	50	13	11	41	*30*
Regional N	*5*	*12*	*16*	*6*	*16*	*19*		*74*

they were not always available. From the resulting subset of 74 countries, or 85 percent of all those I had found to enumerate by ethnicity, I calculated that only a few—six, or 8 percent—actually fell in the first category where mixed identification was impossible (see Table 2.1). In other words, in the overwhelming majority of cases of census ethnic enumeration I observed—92 percent—it was possible to register a mixed identity (although not necessarily the specific group or nomenclature one might prefer). The most common route to such self-identification was through write-in responding: 38 of the ethnicity-enumerating countries, or 51 percent, allowed this approach. However, a sizable share of nations—30, or 41 percent—explicitly provided for mixed identification, usually by offering multi-ethnic response options (i.e. types 3 and 4 above, as opposed to type 2, letting people "mark one or more").

Table 2.1 orders world regions according to their likelihood of explicitly permitting mixed reporting (see the row labeled "Allow Mixed Identification"). Explicit provisions for multiethnic identification were most frequent in South America, North America, and Oceania, and were rare in Europe and Asia.

Accounting for this geographic distribution of mixed-identity reporting is unfortunately beyond the scope of the present chapter. However, its strong association with the Western hemisphere brings at least two factors to mind. One is the role that relatively recent histories of migration play in producing not just intergroup mixture but also official recognition of such mixture. Second is the role that the framing of group differences as "racial" may play. As discussed previously, the term *race* appears almost exclusively on the censuses of former New World slave societies. These are the same societies that nurtured an often-elaborate calculus of racial difference according to fractions of blood quantum; the *casta* paintings of the Spanish colonial world and even English-language terminology like "quadroon" or "half-blood" speak to this (Katzew 2004; Moreno Navarro 1973; Wilson 1992). As a result, the greater tendency to permit contemporary citizens to identify with mixed affiliations may be a legacy of the Americas' racialized understanding of group membership, one where descent is inherited in mathematical fractions of biological essences.

Multiracial classification in cultural context

The widespread opportunity to identify as mixed on censuses that request ethnic information may come as a (welcome) surprise to multiracial people. Yet it is important to be aware that opportunities for multiple-race identification come with constraints. In particular, they are limited by the broader cultural systems of racial conceptualization and classification in which they are embedded. In the comments to follow, I will illustrate these conventions by drawing on the official practices of racial classification in the United States.

Three constraints are of particular importance. First and most fundamentally, the notion of who is multiracial hinges on which groups are perceived to be races in the first place. We might call these "primary" races, like the so-called "primary colours" whose mixture is understood to give rise to the rest of the spectrum.[4] This relationship between multiraciality and racial classification in general is clear when we stop to define what we mean by mixed-race persons. I define multiracial individuals as descendants of two or more groups currently believed to constitute distinct races. In other words, belief about which groups constitute distinct primary races is central for any designation as multiracial. For example, according to the United States' official racial classification standards, Hispanics do not make up a race; they are considered instead to be an ethnic group (Office of Management and Budget 1997). As a result, a person of say Irish and Mexican ancestry is not necessarily a multiracial person, because in this view, Mexican origin does not denote any particular racial membership, and so it does not translate to a racial identity distinct from that of (now-)white Irish descendants. If however the 2020 census comes to include "Hispanic or Latino" among its race categories, then a person who checks off both white and Hispanic as her races will be a mixed-race person from the government's standpoint. Hence the importance of "current belief" in defining multiraciality: being mixed race is not the same in 2010 as it was in 1910, or perhaps as it will be in 2110.

To be more precise, notions of which primary races exist in the world should be understood as one facet of our broader concepts of what race is. Our beliefs about the nature of race—for example, how many races there are and how they are distinct from each other—form complexes that can be labeled *concepts of race* (Morning 2011). And although I have emphasized the role that our ideas about which primary races exist play in our recognition of multiraciality, other understandings of how race works matter too. One example is our model for how racial membership is transmitted across generations. In the United States, the "one-drop rule" dictates that any amount of African ancestry renders an individual racially black (like President Barack Obama), making it difficult to recognize a part-black person as multiracial (Khanna 2010; and see the discussion of "unvalidated" black/white biracial people in Rockquemore and Brunsma 2007). American discussions of multiracial people also tend to rule out individuals with genealogically distant mixed ancestry, excluding African Americans with European ancestry stemming from nineteenth-century intermixture, or Latinos with longstanding European and indigenous roots (Nobles 2000). In short, culturally specific ideas about how race is inherited (in this case via a one-drop rule) and which mixtures are salient (those stemming from recent, voluntary unions as opposed to older, coerced unions in the context of slavery and imperialism) also constrain common thinking about who can or should identify as mixed.

A second major constraint for multiracial reporting, even on censuses that allow it in some way, is that not all types of mixed ancestry have recognized labels or widespread social salience. For example, late nineteenth- and early twentieth-century US censuses included categories for black/white mixture: mulatto, quadroon, and octoroon. They did not, however, provide categories for white/American Indian mixture (though they did furnish enumerators with instructions for such classification—see Morning 2003) or black/Indian mixture.[5] It seems fair to say that while the term "mulatto" was widely familiar, names for black/Indian mixture like "mustee" (Forbes 1993) had less currency and prominence. For historical social and political reasons, certain groups come not only to be understood and therefore labeled as groups (e.g. mulattoes), but also to be subject to interest that encourages broad awareness of their existence. Mulattoes in the nineteenth-century United States straddled the all-important black–white color line and thus were subjects of intense interest in a century where the placement and the meaning of that line was hotly debated. People of black and American Indian ancestry on the other hand received much less attention, as their mixture crossed a boundary line of much less significance for the white majority. Thus official designation as "mulatto" was possible whereas recognition as "mustee" was not.

This historical example is closely related to a third major constraint shaping mixed identification on censuses: nation states make certain identities but not others available for selection on censuses. To return to a contemporary census, the United Kingdom provides for the recognition of certain kinds of racial mixture but not others. The 2001 England and Wales Census enumerates "White and Black Caribbean" people, "White and Black African" respondents, and "White and Asian" inhabitants, but it does not inquire about "Asian and Black Caribbean" people, or "White and Chinese," for example (although it provides a write-in blank). In other words, state interests single out certain kinds of mixed descent for scrutiny, and ignore others. While the relative size of specific mixed groups may partly account for state recognition of specific "mixtures," it is likely to be only one, among various, considerations. As a result, only some kinds of mixedness can be registered in official contexts.

The statistic that most ethnicity-enumerating censuses allow for some kind of multidescent reporting is perhaps misleading. It does not mean that in all such instances, an individual has free rein to identify with the multiracial community of his or her choice. Add to this governmental restraint the underpinning social concepts according to which some kinds of ancestry are perceived as mixed and others are not, and it is clear that our notions and recognition of multiraciality are everywhere embedded in broader and deeper beliefs about racial difference.

One of the significant results of our culturally constructed systems for identifying racial mixture is that the statistics that censuses produce inevitably give us just one slant among many other possible ones on the numbers of people who are mixed race. As Harris and Sim (2002: 625) noted of the 2000 US census, "it was a count of *a* multiracial population, not *the* multiracial population." In the case of the United States, only a fraction of the people who could be considered mixed race are actually designated as such on the decennial census. The 2000 census estimated the multiple-race population at just over 2 percent (Grieco and Cassidy 2001); this, to put it mildly, is just the tip of the iceberg. If we considered the US multiracial population to consist not only of the 2 to 3 percent who identified as such on the 2000 census, but also Latinos and African Americans—three-quarters of whom were already considered by census officials to be mixed race a century ago (US Census Bureau 1918)—as well as whites who report having some American Indian ancestry (or the 20 percent that some scholars argue have non-European ancestry—see Stuckert 1976), we would probably put the share of mixed-race people between 30 and 50 percent of the total US population (Morning 2000).

Conclusion: multiraciality as global phenomenon

The panorama of censuses conducted around the world suggests that the notion of ethnic mixedness is a widespread one. Opportunities to identify with multiple origins however are not unlimited or unconstrained. Local and regional concepts of group difference shape the categories that are socially and officially available, and state interests lead some but not others to be included on census questionnaires. These beliefs and policies are underpinned by broader systems of cultural meaning and social structure. As a consequence, it is clear that we cannot study multiracial people in a vacuum, just as we cannot examine any racially classified group in isolation. To fully understand their experience and circumstances, the larger complex of racial ideology and categorization that is at work in a given society must be taken into account.

Just as comparative research helps identify important features of racial systems in general, it also offers a great deal to the study of multiraciality in particular. First, as the research outlined here shows, comparison draws attention to social or official conventions that are rare or otherwise distinctive. For example, few census questionnaires let respondents express a multiracial identity by combining any primary races they wish; instead, nations generally channel the expression of a mixed identity into a few predetermined categories. Second, this highlighting of particular practices also helps us generate hypotheses about why such approaches have formed, and about the effects they ultimately have. We might ask, for example, what nations that offer "mixed" categories have in common. I have already suggested that the high frequency of explicit multiple-origin options on census questionnaires in the Americas might be related to that hemisphere's relatively high use of "race" as a central ethnic concept. A different kind of inquiry would be to explore the role that the recognition of mixed people might have (or not) in defusing national ethnic tensions.

In closing, I will return to the question I posed at the outset: should we think of mixed-race people as constituting a global community of sorts, or rather as a dispersed collection of separate, more-or-less nation-bound groups? The emphasis I have placed on the culture-specific nature of multiracial classification may suggest that mixed people form local rather than transnational communities. Moreover, there is little evidence to date of a shared consciousness of multiraciality that transcends state borders. Yet it is also clear that, as censuses demonstrate, the social and political awareness of mixedness is fairly widespread throughout the globe. This leaves open a starting point for comparative research on multiraciality, and it signals a potential body of data with which to do it—namely, the demographic information that censuses ultimately collect. These statistics have the potential to reveal how mixed-race populations are changing over time, in terms of both size and other characteristics. If multiracial people come to make up increasing shares of national populations (as seems likely), and acknowledgment of multiraciality grows apace, in the context of an ever more global world we may well witness the future emergence of a transnational consciousness of mixedness.

Notes

1 The author wishes to thank Rosalind Edwards, Alondra Nelson, Wendy Roth, and Miri Song for their helpful comments.
2 Regional groupings are taken from the United Nations Statistical Division, which provided the bulk of the questionnaires in the sample.
3 It is worth noting however that in nations where ethnic affiliations are linked or assigned to individuals through other administrative means (e.g. identity cards, passports), the apparently unconstrained choice offered by the census may in reality be no more than a rehearsal of official categories that individuals are expected to report on multiple occasions.
4 And as Pastoureau (2008) has shown, our notions of which colours are primary are just as historically contingent as our beliefs about principal races.
5 I use the term "American Indian" to refer to the indigenous peoples of North America (and not to Americans of Asian Indian descent).

References

Blum, Alain, and C. Gousseff. 1996. "Statistiques Ethniques et Nationales dans l'Empire Russe et en URSS." Pp. 441–55 in *Démographie et Ethnicité*, edited by J.L. Rallu and Y. Courbage. Paris: INED.

Brunsma, David L. (Ed.). 2006. *Mixed Messages: Multiracial Identities in the "Color-Blind" Era*. Boulder, CO: Lynne Rienner Publishers.

DaCosta, Kimberly McClain. 2007. *Making Multiracials: State, Family, and Market in the Redrawing of the Color Line*. Stanford, CA: Stanford University Press.

Eberhardt, P. 2003. *Ethnic Groups and Population Changes in Twentieth-Century Central-Eastern Europe: History, Data, and Analysis*. Armonk, NY and London: M.E. Sharpe.

Forbes, Jack D. 1993. *Africans and Native Americans: The Language of Race and the Evolution of Red-Black Peoples*. Urbana and Chicago, IL: University of Illinois Press.

Grieco, Elizabeth M., and Rachel C. Cassidy. 2001. *Overview of Race and Hispanic Origin*. Washington, DC: US Department of Commerce.

Gross, Ariela J. 2007. "'Of Portuguese Origin': Litigating Identity and Citizenship Among the Little Races in Nineteenth-Century America." *Law and History Review* 25:467–512.

Harris, David R., and Jeremiah Joseph Sim. 2002. "Who Is Multiracial? Assessing the Complexity of Lived Race." *American Sociological Review* 67 (August):614–27.

Hollinger, David A. 1998. "National Culture and Communities of Descent." *Reviews in American History* 26 (1):312–28.

Katzew, Ilona. 2004. *Casta Painting: Images of Race in Eighteenth-Century Mexico*. New Haven, CT: Yale University Press.

Khanna, Nikki. 2010. "'If You're Half Black, You're Just Black': Reflected Appraisals and the Persistence of the One-Drop Rule." *Sociological Quarterly* 51 (1):96–121.

Lee, Jennifer, and Frank D. Bean. 2004. "America's Changing Color Lines: Immigration, Race/Ethnicity, and Multiracial Identification." *Annual Review of Sociology* 30:221–42.

Marx, Anthony W. 1998. *Making Race and Nation: A Comparison of South Africa, the United States, and Brazil*. Cambridge: Cambridge University Press.

Moreno Navarro, Isidoro. 1973. *Los "Cuadros del Mestizaje Americano": Estudio Antropológico del Mestizaje*. Madrid: Ediciones Jose Porrua Turanzas.

Morning, Ann. 2000. "Who Is Multiracial? Definitions and Decisions." *Sociological Imagination* 37 (4):209–29.

——2003. "New Faces, Old Faces: Counting the Multiracial Population Past and Present." Pp. 41–67 in *New Faces in a Changing America: Multiracial Identity in the 21st Century*, edited by Herman DeBose and Loretta Winters. Thousand Oaks, CA: Sage.

——2008. "Ethnic Classification in Global Perspective: A Cross-National Survey of the 2000 Census Round." *Population Research and Policy Review* 27 (2):239–72.

——2011. *The Nature of Race: How Scientists Think and Teach about Human Difference*. Berkeley, CA: University of California Press.

Nobles, Melissa. 2000. *Shades of Citizenship: Race and the Census in Modern Politics*. Stanford, CA: Stanford University Press.

Office of Management and Budget. 1997. "Revisions to the Standards for the Classification of Federal Data on Race and Ethnicity." *Federal Register*. Washington, DC: Government Printing Office.

Park, Robert E. 1928. "Human Migration and the Marginal Man." *American Journal of Sociology* 33 (6):881–93.

Pastoureau, Michel. 2008. *Noir: Histoire d'une couleur*. Paris: Éditions du Seuil.

Rallu, Jean-Louis, Victor Piché, and Patrick Simon. 2004. "Démographie et Ethnicité: Une Relation Ambiguë." Pp. 481–515 in *Démographie: Analyse et Synthèse*, edited by Graziella Caselli, Jacques Vallin, and Guillaume Wunsch. Paris: Institut National d'Etudes Démographiques.

Rockquemore, Kerry Ann, and David L. Brunsma. 2007. *Beyond Black: Biracial Identity in America*. Lanham, MD: Rowman Littlefield.

Root, Maria P.P. (Ed.). 1996. *The Multiracial Experience: Racial Borders as the New Frontier*. Thousand Oaks, CA: Sage.

Saada, Emmanuelle. 2002. "Race and Sociological Reason in the Republic: Inquiries on the *Métis* in the French Empire (1908–37)." *International Sociology* 17 (3, September):361–91.

Stuckert, Robert P. 1976. "'Race' Mixture: The Black Ancestry of White Americans." Pp. 135–39 in *Physical Anthropology and Archaeology: Introductory Readings*, edited by Peter B. Hammond. New York: Macmillan Publishing Co.

Thompson, Victor. 2006. "A New Take on an Old Idea: Do We Need Multiracial Studies?" *Du Bois Review* 3 (2, Fall):437–47.

US Census Bureau. 1918. *Negro Population 1790–1915*. Washington, DC: Government Printing Office.

Weber, Max. 1978. *Economy and Society*. Berkeley, CA: University of California Press.

Wilson, Terry P. 1992. "Blood Quantum: Native American Mixed Bloods." Pp. 108–25 in *Racially Mixed People in America*, edited by Maria P.P. Root. Newbury Park, CA: Sage.

Winant, Howard. 2001. *The World is a Ghetto: Race and Democracy Since World War II*. New York: Basic Books.

3 Mixed race across time and place

Contrasting Australia with the UK

Ilan Katz

Introduction

The issue of racial mixing has been debated in the academic literature and in the political domain for centuries. Over the vast majority of this period the arguments against racial mixing have been put forward by conservatives, who have argued that mixing of races and cultures is 'unnatural', 'morally wrong', damaging to the individuals concerned and undermining of society as a whole. Progressives have historically tended to argue that racial mixing is a natural part of the human condition and that it should be encouraged because it demonstrates a tolerance for diversity and racial harmony. However in the UK during the 1980s the debate changed, and for the first time it was progressives who were arguing against mixing and (relatively conservative) liberals who argued in favour of racial and cultural mixing. This new configuration has now become the dominant discourse although the debate is no longer as polarised as it was at that time, and some accommodation has taken place between the two viewpoints.

Although the arguments on both sides of the debate tend to be made in universalist terms (e.g. that racial mixing will always cause identity problems, or conversely racial mixing is a sign of good inter-communal relations and mental health), this chapter will show that in reality these debates are bound by both chronology and geography and that in different times and places even the basic terms 'race' and 'mixing' have different connotations and implications. The chapter will particularly draw on the situation in Australia to demonstrate the contingent nature of arguments about identity and its role in the wider discourse on race. A key aim of this chapter is to contribute to the question of how the wider social and historical context relates to the day-to-day experiences of individuals who are racially mixed, and the extent to which mixed-race people and inter-racial families can be seen as reflecting the broader society in which they are living.

Recent debates on mixed race in the UK

Race and racism have been concerns of social policy over many decades, but the 1980s saw a new dimension to this issue in social policy in the UK, and particularly in the delivery of social welfare to children. The 1980s saw the emergence of anti-discrimination and anti-racism as key objectives of social welfare, and previous ideologies, in particular the 'colour blind' approach (which at the time were viewed as progressive policies aimed at combating the racist ideologies which were prevalent), were now seen as being reactionary and counter-productive.

The debate around mixed-race children was played out mainly in the social work arena and was closely tied in with the much more emotive debates around trans-racial and inter-country adoption, because both involved the development of identity of 'black' children in 'white' families. The issue was debated as a political and social question but was mainly focused on the psychological problems which were assumed to emerge for the children concerned. In particular contention was the issue of whether a 'racially' mixed child would by definition be psychologically 'mixed up', and whether the only way of avoiding psychological damage was to ensure that mixed-race children grew up with a strong sense of black identity. A major characteristic of this argument is that it took 'essentialism' to the extreme. 'Black' and 'white' were treated as mutually exclusive and inviolable categories, and every individual had to be assigned to one of these categories.

However a few empirical studies in the 1980s and early 1990s, including most significantly those of Barbara Tizard and Ann Phoenix (1993) (as well as my own work (Katz, 1996)), showed that the reality was far more complex than these representations allowed for. 'Racial' mixing occurred in a multitude of different ways, with a huge array of different racial combinations. Identity and identity development turned out not to be monolithic or linear, but are fluid, contradictory and complex. It was this insight that eventually fractured the essentialist model of anti-racism which has since been replaced by multiculturalism and diversity. One of the features of both sides of this debate is that it tends to conflate descriptive or empirical evidence with ethical or moral considerations; that is to confuse what mixed-race people actually feel about themselves with beliefs about what they should feel.

Identity is now understood to be a process involving constant interactions between individuals and their environments. It is therefore not a fixed state, but is contingent on the characteristics of the individual, his or her immediate environment and the wider social context. Moreover people can develop a variety of identity positions without necessarily suffering psychological harm. Nevertheless, the diversity, mixedness and hybridity of society does not imply that identity is infinitely fluid, nor that identities can be consciously chosen. The context constrains identities and even forces people into identities which they have not preferred and sometimes never even acknowledged. Thus identity is not just a mask or persona or a suit on a department store clothes rack that one can simply pick and wear. Each person has a narrow range of identities from which to choose, and the context determines that range.

Much of the early research and theorising on race, racial mixing and marginalisation in the UK was drawn from the USA, despite the very different situations regarding race and migration in the two countries. The arguments were also influenced by French anti-colonial theorists such as Frantz Fanon.[1] This gave the debate an international and timeless flavour rather than being viewed as a struggle which was being waged in a particular socio-historical context. However it has turned out that although there are deep resonances within the debate which apply wherever marginality and hybridity occur as part of the human condition, there were (and are) important aspects of this debate which are contingent on particular social and historical contexts. Even the basic terms of the debate 'race' and 'mixed' are quite different both over time and in different places.[2]

In this chapter I will explore in more depth how the wider social, geographical and political context can bear on the range of available identities for people of 'mixed race', and how the very notions of 'mixed race', mixed heritage, biraciality and other designations are all reflective of specific social, political and cultural developments in particular times and places.

Australia

The case of Australia offers an interesting contrast to the situation in the UK. Australia is socially, culturally and politically very similar to the UK. Indeed a large proportion of the Australian population is British by birth or at least has British (or Irish) parents or grandparents. However Australia (like Canada and New Zealand, and the USA) has to address issues relating not only to migrant minority ethnic groups, but also to the Indigenous or First Nation populations. Both of these issues have created ongoing challenges for social policy ever since Australia was originally settled, and both continue to be highly contentious policy arenas.

Indigenous Australians

The history of relationships between white settlers and the Indigenous population of Australia (Aboriginal Australians and Torres Strait Islanders) is characterised by conflict, violence and tension. Unlike New Zealand and Canada, both of which have signed treaties with their Indigenous populations, Australia does not recognise its First Nations constitutionally and has never signed such a treaty. Indeed, to this very day, the Australian constitution contains the following text:

> Australian Constitution – Section 25 – Provisions as to races disqualified from voting:
>
> For the purposes of the last section, if by the law of any State all persons of any race are disqualified from voting at elections for the more numerous House of the Parliament of the State, then, in reckoning the number of the people of the State or of the Commonwealth, persons of the race resident in that State shall not be counted.
>
> (Commonwealth of Australia, 1900)

Policy towards the Indigenous population has moved between open hostility, paternalism, protection, integration, self-determination, 'practical reconciliation' and 'tough love'. All of these policy positions have had damaging effects on the Indigenous population who have, as a result, suffered 'generational trauma'.[3] Indigenous Australians continue to be the most disadvantaged group in Australian society, with lower socioeconomic status, shorter life expectancy, higher rates of incarceration and lower levels of education than the non-Indigenous population (Australian Bureau of Statistics, 2010).

One of the most traumatic chapters in Aboriginal history relates to the events surrounding the 'Stolen Generations', which still cast a long shadow over many Aboriginal families and over relationships between the Indigenous population and the Australian government. The Stolen Generations refers to a deliberate policy of the Australian government, together with churches and NGOs, in which 'half-caste' children were forcibly removed and placed in white institutions and families with the ultimate aim of 'breeding out' the Indigenous population. These removals lasted from the early part of the twentieth century until the 1960s. The traumatic stories of the victims of the Stolen Generations were finally made public in the Bringing Them Home report which was published by the Australian Human Rights and Equal Opportunities Commission after an in-depth inquiry (HREOC, 1997). The inquiry was set up under the Keating Labor Government, but reported when the new Liberal (conservative) government came into power, and their response was to contest the accuracy of the report's findings and to reject the need for apology. Ten years later when Kevin Rudd was elected, he finally apologised to the Aboriginal community for the Stolen Generations in his first act shortly after becoming prime minister of Australia in December 2007.

Indigenous Australians were also subject to strict racial classification, which created sad and ridiculous anomalies as illustrated by the following narrative:

> In 1935 a fair-skinned Australian of part-indigenous descent was ejected from a hotel for being an Aboriginal. He returned to his home on the mission station to find himself refused entry because he was not an Aboriginal. He tried to remove his children but was told he could not because they were Aboriginal. He walked to the next town where he was arrested for being an Aboriginal vagrant and placed on the local reserve. During the Second World War he tried to enlist but was told he could not because he was Aboriginal. He went interstate and joined up as a non-Aboriginal. After the war he could not acquire a passport without permission because he was Aboriginal. He received exemption from the Aborigines Protection Act – and was told that he could no longer visit his relations on the reserve because he was not an Aboriginal. He was denied permission to enter the Returned Servicemen's Club because he was.
>
> (Gardiner-Garden, 2000 quoting Peter Read, 1996: 3)

As a response to this history there is a very strong culture in Australia of downplaying the racial mixing of Indigenous Australians. Policy has shifted radically so that anyone who self-identifies as Aboriginal or Torres Strait Islander, and is accepted by the Indigenous community, is considered Indigenous. The census relies on self-identification.

The New South Wales Aboriginal Land Rights Act 1983 (New South Wales Parliament, 1983) defines as 'Aboriginal' as anyone who:

(a) is a member of the Aboriginal race of Australia,
(b) identifies as an Aboriginal, and
(c) is accepted by the Aboriginal community as an Aboriginal.

This deliberately removes colour from the definition, and was a response to the previous racist regime of classifying Aboriginal Australians (similarly to American slaves), as Quadroons, Octoroons and so on (Maddison, 2009) or conversely of the 'one drop' notion which was notoriously used in the USA to disinherit slave owners' descendents, and was similarly used in Australia to disinherit the children of white farm owners and pastoralists.

Although there may be divisions along colour lines within the Indigenous community, they are all identified in political and social discourse as 'black' or 'blackfellas' irrespective of their physical colour. Nevertheless being an Indigenous Australian is not just a matter of identifying as Aboriginal or Torres Strait Islander. Aboriginal Australians have strong obligations and associations with 'country' (i.e. the particular area for whom their nation or clan is the traditional custodian) and with their specific nation and clan. Thus identifying as Indigenous is not arbitrary or only a matter of individual choice – it is embedded and prescribed by a range of social relationships and obligations.

Because of the particular history, therefore, classifications of the Indigenous and white settler populations in Australia are dichotomous; all Indigenous Australians are defined (politically) as 'black' and all non-Indigenous Australians are by definition 'white'. This is irrespective of their own personal feelings and identifications as well as their physical colour.[4] Nevertheless this political identification is still controversial. At the time of writing this chapter there is a trial underway in the Australian Federal Court in Melbourne in which a right-wing newspaper reporter and blogger, Andrew Bolt, is being sued by five prominent 'light-skinned' Indigenous Australians. In a series of articles Bolt accused these people (and others) of claiming Aboriginal identity in order to further their own careers and to gain materially (Bolt, 2009). One of the points being raised in the trial is how 'black' an individual has to be to legitimately identify as Aboriginal.

In summary, although the identity of Indigenous Australians is not contested officially, and there are no 'mixed' Indigenous Australians, the question of identity is still an important issue in the civil discourse, and is to some extent still influenced by public policy.

Migration policy

Australia has also had a complex and difficult policy with regard to migration. The country has, since settlement, always relied on the influx of large numbers of migrants to remain economically viable. For many years the migration policy was governed by the maxim 'populate or perish'. Nevertheless there is a history of xenophobia and racism in Australia as there is in all colonial countries, and Australia has a shameful history in this respect – in some ways even worse than South Africa (Welsh, 2004). For many years immigration was regulated by the 'White Australia' policy framework. This policy began in the early years of the twentieth century shortly after federation, and persisted until after the Second World War. At that time immigration was largely limited to British and Irish nationals. In the late 1940s immigrants from southern Europe began to flow in as a result of acute labour shortages after the war. It is only since the 1970s that Asians and other non-Westerners have been allowed to emigrate to Australia in any numbers (Jupp, 2007). In the 1970s the official policy changed to 'Multiculturalism', which has had a rather rocky policy ride in Australia (Jupp, 1997) but which has just about continued to be official government policy. Now Australia is one of the most multicultural countries in the world with almost a third of the population having a parent born overseas. Migration, especially that of asylum seekers, is an important and continuing political issue which often attracts media attention (Katz & Redmond, 2010). Table 3.1 below gives an overview of how policy towards Indigenous Australians and migrants and minorities has co-evolved since settlement. There are some points of coherence – most notably the

Table 3.1 Australian policy timeline: Indigenous and migrant/minority

Period	*Indigenous*	*Migration/Minority*
1800–1900	**Terra nullius**: From 1788 Australia was taken over by British colonists on the premise that the land belonged to no one. In other words according to the colonists, Aboriginal people were incapable of owning the land and had no recognisable form of sovereignty and so this justified the taking of lands.	States have different migration policies but none allow non-white migrants. Workers from Pacific Islands forcibly recruited but not allowed to settle.
1900 Federation	Indigenous people not classified as citizens in the constitution and not counted in census.	White Australia policy – only British, Irish and NZ migrants allowed to settle.
1900s–1930s	**Protection**: Indigenous people were moved onto reserves or missions. A large part of the Aboriginal population was segregated.	White Australia policy continues.

Table 3.1 (continued)

Period	*Indigenous*	*Migration/Minority*
	Stolen generations: From as early as 1871 in Victoria, and across all States and Territories by the early 1900s, Aboriginal children were forcibly removed from their families and communities to the care of non-Aboriginal people with the aim of assimilating them into non-Aboriginal society.	
1930s–1950s	**Assimilation**: In 1937 the Commonwealth Government determined that Aboriginal people 'not of full blood' should be assimilated into the broader population.	**Populate or Perish**: Immigration encouraged from UK and Ireland. Some children removed from families forcibly. After WW2 immigrants began arriving from Italy, Greece etc.
1960s	**The 1967 Referendum**: Held to amend the Constitution to allow Indigenous peoples to be included in the national census and to give federal Parliament the power to make laws in relation to Indigenous people. **Equal pay**: In 1965 Aboriginal stockmen were granted equal wages.	
1970s–1980s	**Land rights**: In 1976, the federal government passed land rights law for Indigenous peoples in the Northern Territory. Most states also have some form of Land Rights legislation.	Large-scale migration from Lebanon and Vietnam, migrants begin to come from many other countries. Multiculturalism takes over from White Australia policy. *Racial Discrimination Act 1975* passed.
1990s–2007	**The Northern Territory Intervention**: In 2007 the Howard Government announced a national emergency response to protect Aboriginal children in the Northern Territory from sexual abuse and family violence. The 12 measures announced were exempt from the application of the Racial Discrimination Act 1975.	**Clampdown on asylum seekers**: Howard government restricts asylum seekers, wins 2001 election partly because of immigration fears. Multiculturalism dropped as official policy in favour of citizenship. However migration continues to grow.
Now	**The Apology**: In 2008 Kevin Rudd apologised for the 'Stolen Generations'.	2011 re-commitment of the government to multiculturalism.

strenuous efforts over a century until the end of the Second World War to keep Australia as a homogenous white Anglo-Celtic society. However it is notable that these are considered to be separate policy domains in Australia. Although Indigenous and Multicultural affairs were for some time co-located in the same government department, they were never part of a coherent policy response to minorities, and different policy structures have always been in place to address the issues in these communities.

Because of its history and its geographical location, Australia has very few migrants who would be classified as 'black' in the UK context. The main sources of migration have been the UK and New Zealand, followed by Greece, Italy and Eastern Europe, Lebanon, Vietnam, China and South East Asia, and the Pacific Islands. In the past decade substantial numbers of people from East Africa, Afghanistan, Iraq and Sri Lanka have arrived in Australia as refugees.

Although the idea of a 'White Australia' was a key factor in the development of Australian national identity, the concept of 'race' has deliberately been excluded from the official lexicon in Australia in recent years. When the 'White Australia' policy was eventually abandoned, it was superseded by the official adoption of 'multiculturalism' and more recently 'citizenship' (Koleth, 2010). British terms such as 'BME' (Black and Minority Ethnic), 'visible minority' or 'minority ethnic' are not used, and minority/migrant groups have been labelled respectively 'NESB' (Non English Speaking Background), 'LOTE' (Language Other Than English (spoken in the home)) or more commonly 'CALD' (Culturally and Linguistically Diverse), but never 'ethnic' or 'racial'. The opposite of CALD is 'Anglo-Australian' or 'Anglo-Celtic',[5] not 'white'. CALD includes not only people of Chinese and Somalian heritage, but also those of Swedish and Italian origin, and is therefore not even a good designation for people of colour or visible minorities. Nevertheless it is often used as a rather poor proxy for disadvantage and minority status (Sawrikar & Katz, 2009).

On the one hand, whilst CALD groups are often identified collectively, they are also classified with 'Anglo' in contrast to Indigenous, and most official reports either ignore them altogether or still classify them by country of origin (e.g. families where at least one parent is born overseas), or language. On the other hand Australia is much more open about discussions of minority groups than the UK. For example police and the media will often mention people of 'Middle Eastern' or 'Pacific islander' appearance, and minorities are identified in the media in ways which in the UK would be considered discriminatory. Nevertheless all official categorisations in Australia are by cultural or religious affiliation or country of origin, and there is no official way of differentiating visible or 'racial' minorities.

This has left very little space for any sort of 'racial' identity in Australia, in particular mixed-race or mixed (racial) heritage. However because of the lack of official recognition there is relatively little research on experiences, attainments and wellbeing of CALD people generally and mixed-race Australians in particular. Indeed the non-recognition makes this sector of the population very hard to identify.

One of the few accounts in the literature of the mixed-race experience is provided by Maureen Perkins (a British-born mixed-race person), who has written poignantly about how this plays out for 'brown' people in Australia:

> My culture is Anglo (dominant in Australia), but my skin is brown. I am neither black, nor white. Somehow this places me in an unspeakable position in Australian society, which can only conceptualize either Aboriginal, non-Aboriginal (white) or ethnic immigrant ... Those who do experience this marginalization joke about the 'where do you come from?' question. This is the one which means that the questioner wants to know why you are coloured, but doesn't dare to ask. Underlying the question ... is the supposition of the multiracial person's foreignness ... Thus, when the answer 'Australia' is given, the supplementary question follows: 'No, where do you really come from?' The assumption, of course, is that there is no such thing as a brown Australian.
>
> (Perkins, 2004, p. 194)

Many of the themes identified by Perkins are familiar from the international literature on mixed-race identity, and it is fair to assume that in many ways, on a personal level, the issues faced by mixed-race Australians are probably very similar to those in the UK or USA. The few anecdotal studies of racial and cultural mixing include mixes which would not in British terms be considered as 'mixed race' or 'mixed heritage' at all. For example Penny and Khoo's (1996) study of mixed marriages included American/Australian, Dutch/Australian and Italian/Australian families, as well as more familiar 'racial' mixes such as Australian/Indonesian and Australian/Vietnamese. Penny and Khoo did not find that intermarriage in itself produced high levels of marital unhappiness or psychological distress, especially when the marriage had been entered into for 'positive' purposes (i.e. the partners loved each other) rather than negative purposes (to obtain a visa, legitimise a child or compensate for a loss). However a number of couples had experienced some discrimination.

Another significant development in Australia in the past decade has been the rise of the importance of religion, rather than race or culture, as the primary site of division amongst the population. This is primarily the result of 9/11 and the events subsequent to it (for Australia in particular the Bali bombings of 2004 and 2006) and the so called 'clash of civilisations'. In Australia, like the rest of the developed world, this has had the effect of 'othering' Muslims, and consequently reducing the 'otherness' of people from other religious backgrounds, irrespective of their racial origins. This change has had an enormous impact on the Muslim population in Australia, one of the consequences being that whereas they had previously identified (at least socially) more with their country of origin or linguistic group, they now see themselves primarily as Muslim Australians – a category which simply did not exist in the public consciousness before 9/11 (Pe-Pua, Gendera, Katz & O'Connor, 2010). Interestingly in my own research in the UK carried out in the 1980s, Muslim/non-Muslim mixes stood out as being particularly challenging for families because the religion required Muslims to follow a particular lifestyle, and to raise their children in the Muslim tradition which is not compatible with 'mixing'. These families tended to resolve the tension by the non-Muslim partner converting to Islam (Katz, 1996). However at that time these issues were not considered politically or socially significant, especially if the partners were from the same 'race'. Rather they were considered to be personal issues to be resolved privately along with a range of cultural and other differences which could arise within families.

Comparing Australia and the UK

Australia and the UK are comparable in many respects; their political institutions are similar, the dominant language and culture is similar and even the political debates around topics such as race and immigration are very alike. However, there are some important differences relevant to the identity of mixed-race people. Importantly Australia differs from the UK in that there is a strong patriotic culture and a strong identification with being 'Australian'. The specific history of colonisation and migration in Australia has fundamentally affected the way policies about race in general and mixed race in particular has played out. Whereas in the UK (and the USA) mixed-race/biracial/mixed-heritage people have increasingly been recognised as a social group by both policy makers and academics, in Australia they continue to be ignored in public policy and academia. This analysis has shown that the lack of recognition is not merely an oversight by policy makers and academics but is rather a factor of the broader context of race relations in Australia which has been dominated by relations between the settler population and the Indigenous Australians on the one hand, and by the history of immigration, particularly the 'White Australia' policies on the other.

There are a number of important questions raised by comparing the situation of mixed-race people in Australia with those in the UK. Perhaps the most significant question relates to whether and how these differences in policy and cultural context impact on individuals and their identity formation. To what extent does official recognition of 'mixed race' as a social policy issue, rather than as a personal or familial concern, bear on the day-to-day lives of people of mixed race and their families? What is the impact of the designation 'black' being primarily associated with Indigenous Australians on the lives of other visible minorities, particularly people of mixed race?

There is no empirical evidence which directly links the lived experience of individuals and families with the designations and categories used by officials or government agencies. At the personal level, identity is likely to be far more influenced by relationships within the nuclear and extended family, the local community, school and so on. However the real issue is how these day-to-day interactions are influenced (or not influenced) by the broader social milieu and in particular by the policy context of different countries. There is no real information about whether Australians of mixed racial heritage are more or less likely than Britons to identify as 'mixed', attempt to 'pass as white' or identify as 'black', nor whether they are more or less likely to be marginalised and excluded by their peers and others around them.

Official categorisations and designations probably make little direct difference to the lives of individuals in and of themselves, and it is possible that they are confined to the bureaucratic and administrative domains. However it would be surprising if these national contexts did not influence, perhaps very subtly, the interactions between parents and their children, and between families and the broader social ecology. Recognition of one's situation in the media and in public discourse are likely to have important effects on self concept and relationships. It is certainly clear that negative media or political attention on one's group can have profound effects for identity development, as I have noted above in relation to Muslims (and also asylum seekers), and the corollary – that positive depictions in the media will positively affect some forms of identification – is also likely.

Conclusion

The analysis presented in this chapter shows that there is both continuity and discontinuity in the way mixed-race people have been treated by policy makers and in the academic literature over time and place. Some of the elements of the discourse – resistance to or embracing of miscegenation and hybridity, and the prevalence of racial prejudice against visible minorities, are constants in most societies and over most of history. However 'racial' identity and its development are not essential human qualities, and are intimately associated with the immediate context in which the child is being brought up, which is in turn affected by changing political, cultural and demographic factors.

The fluid and ever-changing nature of identity and mixedness does not mean, however, that identities themselves can be consciously chosen, nor that the range of available identities for any individual is infinite. Each era and each national context opens up new possible identities but also closes down other viable identities. Unconscious and conscious identifications and emotional attachments make it difficult to easily move from one identity to another. For example a person in Australia who describes her identity as 'mixed race' or 'mixed heritage' is likely to be met with confusion or misunderstanding, as these are not terms used in common discourse.

Nevertheless the context now is much more conducive to mixedness in a number of different ways. It is possible that mixed-race people in the UK (and perhaps even in Australia) will eventually form a new and separate social group with its own identity or even its own traditions and culture, such as those of the Métis in Canada, the Coloureds in South Africa or the Creoles of various countries.

The tensions underlying policy and practice in this area are likely to continue and perhaps even exacerbate. On the one hand any attempt to segment the population on a racial, religious or cultural basis will inevitably result in unintended consequences for groups at the margins and will leave certain sectors of the population in an ill-defined 'grey area'. On the other hand attempts to include everybody will inevitably result in the denial of strongly held identifications and will deny some people their heritage. In Australia there is still some way to go to even recognise that 'racial' mixedness is an issue for social policy.

We must also be mindful of the ecological fallacy. It may be feasible, or even desirable, for minority groups in society to band together and form political alliances (e.g. 'black' and 'Muslim'). However these political groupings do not necessarily translate into the personal identities of individuals who are designated as members of that particular group. Nor is it necessarily the case that an individual who has a dual (or multiple) heritage from groups who are in conflict will necessarily be psychologically conflicted or 'mixed up'.

Thus mixing, mixedness and miscegenation will persist and will continue to challenge the mainstream. Every new generation is likely to bring new realities which will undermine what are considered universal and unchangeable categories.

Notes

1 Fanon's incisive analysis of inter-racial relationships *Black Skin, White Masks* (Fanon, 1967 [1952]) examined how personal and sexual relationships between black and white people are dominated by the unconscious internalisation of colonialist ideologies which represented white people as powerful and resourceful whereas black people are represented as submissive and accommodating.
2 For example in Germany policy makers and practitioners have been extremely reluctant to use the term 'race' at all – it could be interpreted as referring back to the Nazi era. They use the term 'binational' and it includes Italian/Germans, Turkish/Germans and other Europeans (Frieben-Blum, Jacobs & Wiessmeier, 2001).
3 A good summary of the history of Indigenous policy and its effect on Indigenous families is available from the Australian Human Rights Commission http://www.hreoc.gov.au/bth/taken/track_the_history.html (retrieved 3.1.12).
4 The Indigenous population of Australia in fact contains a wide diversity of 'mixtures' not only with the Anglo-Celtic majority but also with migrants from many parts of the world (O'Reilly, 1994), and thus cannot be categorised simply by the degree of 'white' or 'black' in their ancestry.
5 Interestingly the term 'Anglo-Celtic' has been criticised by some commentators, for example Patrick O'Farrell (1992) who points out that the English and Irish immigrants had very different migration experiences in Australia and formed socially different groups. Indeed, the term 'mixed' or 'mixed marriage' referred to Protestant/Catholic marriages which were very strongly opposed by both sides (McHugh, 2009).

References

Australian Bureau of Statistics. (2010). 'The health and welfare of Australia's Aboriginal and Torres Strait Islander peoples.' Retrieved 3.1.12 from http://www.abs.gov.au/AUSSTATS/abs@.nsf/lookup/4704.0Main+Features12010.

Bolt, A. (2009, 1.4.2011). 'White is the new black.' Retrieved 3.1.12 from http://blogs.news.com.au/heraldsun/andrewbolt/index.php/heraldsun/column_white_is_the_new_black.

Commonwealth of Australia (1900). Commonwealth of Australia Constitution Act (1900).

Fanon, F. (1967 [1952]). *Black Skin, White Masks.* New York: Grove Press.

Frieben-Blum, E., Jacobs, K., & Wiessmeier, B. (2001). *Wer ist Fremd: Ethnische Herkunft, Familie und Gesellschaft* (*Who Is Foreign? Ethnic Origin, Family and Society*). Berlin: Leske und Budric.

Gardiner-Garden, J. (2000). 'Research Note 18 2000–01: the definition of Aboriginality (Vol. 2009).' Canberra: Parliament of Australia.

HREOC. (1997). *Bringing Them Home: Report of the National Inquiry into the Separation of Aboriginal and Torres Strait Islander Children from Their Families.* Canberra: Human Rights and Equal Opportunities Commission.

Jupp, J. (1997). 'Immigration and national identity: multiculturalism.' In G. Stokes (ed.), *The Politics of Identity in Australia* (pp. 132–57). Melbourne: Cambridge University Press.

——(2007). *From White Australia to Woomera: The Story of Australian Immigration.* Sydney: Cambridge University Press.

Katz, I. (1996). *The Construction of Racial Identity in Children of Mixed Parentage: Mixed Metaphors.* London; Philadelphia, PA: J. Kingsley Publishers.

Katz, I., & Redmond, G. (2010). 'Review of the circumstances among children in immigrant families in Australia.' *Child Indicators Research*, 3(4), 439–58.

Koleth, E. (2010). 'Research Paper 6 2010–11: multiculturalism: a review of Australian policy statements and recent debates in Australia and overseas'. Canberra: Parliament of Australia.

McHugh, S. (2009). 'How the Irish rose above Australia's social apartheid.' *Sydney Morning Herald*, 14 October: www.smh.com.au/opinion/society-and-culture/how-the-Irish-rose-above-Australias-social-apartheid-20091014-gvyg.html#ixzz1jTiN6GHK. Accessed 12.1.2012.

Maddison, S. (2009). *Black Politics: Inside the Complexity of Aboriginal Political Culture.* Sydney: Allen & Unwin.

New South Wales Parliament (1983). Aboriginal Land Rights Act (1983).

O'Farrell, P. (1992). *The Catholic Church and Community: An Australian History.* Revised 3rd edition. Kensington: University of New South Wales Press.

O'Reilly, J. (1994). 'Demographic implications of Aboriginal out-marriage.' *Journal of Population Research*, 11(2), 149–57.

Pe-Pua, R., Gendera, S., Katz, I., & O'Connor, A. (2010). *Meeting the Needs of Australian Muslim Families: Exploring Marginalisation, Family Issues and 'Best Practice' in Service Provision.* Sydney: Social Policy Research Centre, University of New South Wales.

Penny, J., & Khoo, S.-E. (1996). *Intermarriage: A Study of Migration and Integration.* Canberra: Bureau of Immigration, Multicultural and Population Research.

Perkins, M. (2004). 'Australian mixed race.' *European Journal of Cultural Studies*, 7(2), 177–99.

Sawrikar, P., & Katz, I. (2009). 'How useful is the term 'Culturally and Linguistically Diverse' (CALD) in Australian research, practice, and policy discourse?' Paper presented at the Australian Social Policy Conference. Retrieved 3.1.12 from http://www.sprc.unsw.edu.au/media/File/Paper276.pdf.

Tizard, B., & Phoenix, A. (1993). *Black, White, or Mixed Race? Race and Racism in the Lives of Young People.* London: Routledge.

Welsh, F. (2004). *Great Southern Land: A New History of Australia.* London: Penguin/Allen Lane.

4 From 'Draughtboard Alley' to 'Brown Britain'

The 'ordinariness' of racial mixing and mixedness in British society[1]

Chamion Caballero

Introduction

In Jennifer Worth's popular novel about life as a midwife in the East End of London in the 1950s, she talks about the difficulty that men faced before DNA testing in knowing for certain that any children were theirs – unless, she says, the child was of a different race:

> If a husband happens to be fathering another man's child, he is not likely to know and, as they say, 'what the eye does not see, the heart does not grieve over'. But what happens when his wife brings forth a black man's child? The East Enders had hardly faced this before, but after the Second World War the potential was there.
>
> (Worth 2002: 246)

Yet, contrary to Worth's perception, racial mixing and mixedness were not uncommon in Britain before the Second World War. Indeed, in Canning Town, only a few miles east from the heart of the London Docklands where Worth was a midwife, a black population mostly made up of sailors had settled and raised families with local white women during the early twentieth century. Many of these were residents of 'Draughtboard Alley', so called because of the number of black and white families who lived alongside each other (Bourne 2001: 38).

Whilst over the past few decades, mixed-race people, couples and families in Britain have become increasingly visible in the public eye, there is still a tendency to herald their presence as part of a new multicultural phenomenon – what has been dubbed the rise of 'Beige' or 'Brown Britain'.[2] Yet, such groups have a long presence in Britain, as evidenced not only by late eighteenth- and early twentieth-century public debates about the implications of interracial relationships and 'mulattoes' or 'half-caste' children but also, as is slowly being revealed, through their own accounts.

Drawing on findings from a British Academy-funded project,[3] this chapter examines the intersection between the perceptions of officialdom with those of mixed-race people, couples and families themselves. Concentrating on the period between 1920 and 1950, it discusses the experiences of these groups in what might be considered the 'era of moral condemnation' for racial mixing and mixedness. Indeed, during this time the stigmatisation of mixed-race people and families in Britain appears at its greatest, a process to which many major institutions and significant public figures contributed.

Certainly, over these three decades, and from all quarters, rang constant admonitions of the psychological and social dangers of crossing racialised boundaries, accompanied by often visceral reactions to such transgressions. Yet, despite the warnings of violence, ostracism, hostility and isolation, women and men in Britain still actively and habitually crossed racial boundaries and formed relationships and families. Indeed, certain neighbourhoods in Britain, particularly port communities such as Tiger Bay in Cardiff and Toxteth in Liverpool were, as Tabili (1996: 187) notes, 'sustained by interracial family networks' with mixing and mixedness a commonplace, even typical occurrence. Alongside the more familiar tales of social bigotry and prejudice facing mixed-race couples, families and people can thus also be glimpsed threads of tolerance, acceptance and inclusion and, most importantly, a sense of everyday 'ordinariness' largely ignored in the history of this group to date.

Official and institutional views of racial mixing and mixedness

Longstanding and widespread as racial mixing and mixedness in Britain has been, so too has been a sense of problematisation. In 1772, Edward Long, the British colonial administrator and historian complained that:

> The lower class of women in England, are remarkably fond of the blacks, for reasons too brutal to mention; they would connect themselves with horses and asses if the laws permitted them. By these ladies, they generally have a numerous brood … This is a venomous and dangerous ulcer, that threatens to disperse its malignancy far and wide, until every family catches infection from it.
>
> (quoted in Fryer 1984: 157–58)

While such sentiments on racial mixing were commonly shared by many of Long's contemporaries and inevitably flourished under the racial imperialism of the nineteenth century (Lorimer 1978), the twentieth century saw these types of objection crystallise into a more pervasive and focused public discourse. The demand for civilian and military labour during the First World War saw Britain draw on its Empire for resources and, as such, its minority ethnic population once more began to increase and settle. This, largely male, population was diverse in both its racial and ethnic constitution, as well as its occupation: it contained not only sailors and soldiers, but also students, merchants, entertainers, sportsmen and aristocrats (Green 2000). Alongside the war's creation of a surplus of white British women of marriageable age, many of whom had become economically and socially independent (Bland 2005), thus came distinct opportunities – across society – for racial mixing between these groups.[4]

As such, fear of 'miscegenation' during the 1920s and 1930s was rife; even the briefest glance at commentaries by academics, politicians, policymakers and other institutional forces during this period reveals the extensive nature of their moral concern and condemnation. The 1919 race riots – in which a series of violent disturbances targeting black, Arab and other minorities occurred in nine of Britain's main ports after the demobilisation of First World War service personnel – were not only the result of anger and resentment at 'coloured' men 'taking' white men's jobs but also 'their' women (Ansari 2004; Bland 2005; Seed 2006). Certainly, the media, police officials and other dignitaries, such as the former British colonial administrator, Sir Ralph Williams, blamed these interracial relationships for causing the violence (Bland 2005; Balachandran 2011), Williams writing to *The Times* in 1919 that 'sexual relations between white women and coloured men revolt our very nature … What blame … to those white men who, seeing the conditions and loathing them, resort to violence?' (quoted in Fryer 1984: 311).

Such tensions persisted throughout the 1920s in cities across Britain; in 1929, an official of the British Council for the Welfare of the Mercantile Marine reported that in Cardiff and Manchester 'difficulties are increasing in connection with the association of coloured seamen with white women'. To prevent this 'demoralising development', the Chief Constable of Cardiff suggested the desirability of adopting the South African model and bringing anti-miscegenation laws into Britain (quoted in Banton 1953: 80). There had been earlier attempts to curb such 'developments': in 1924, the Foreign Office had added 'Chinese' to its warning statement provided to British women by marriage registrars which, already operating in relation to 'Hindus, Moslems, African Negroes, etc.', advised British women of the legal dangers of marrying 'aliens' (Bland 2005: 45–46).[5]

Rich (1990) adeptly demonstrates how these 'constantly voiced concerns' regarding racial mixing by British politicians, police and other high-ranking public officials gradually widened by the 1930s from a focus on interracial relationships to the issue of 'half-caste' children. Marie Stopes, the family planning pioneer, was a fierce opponent of interracial relationships, advocating that all half-castes should be 'sterilised at birth' (Hall 1977: 182), an opinion perhaps less surprising to modern readers when considering that Stopes was a prominent eugenicist. Concerned with promoting awareness of hereditary qualities and encouraging social responsibility to improving the human race by these ends (Mazumdar 1991), eugenics propagandists tended to be highly concerned about the effects of 'race crossing' on society; Ruggles Gates – the first husband of Marie Stopes – stated in the 1920s Eugenics Review that it commonly resulted in 'disharmony of physical, mental and temperamental qualities' (quoted in Bland 2007: 68).

With eugenics enthusiastically embraced by scientists, politicians, intellectuals and social reformers across the political spectrum (Dikötter 1998), it is hardly surprising that concern regarding this 'disharmony' increasingly began to feature in public debate. In port cities in the late 1920s, authorities were becoming greatly 'worried' about children from mixed relationships; officials in Cardiff, for example, cautioned that racial mixing had seen 'the consequent growth of a half-caste population, alien in sentiment and habits to the native white inhabitants' (quoted in Banton 1953: 80). Similar warnings were touted vociferously in the media. In 1929 the *Daily Herald* declared that 'hundreds of half-caste children with vicious tendencies' were 'growing up in Cardiff as the result of black men mating with white women' whilst in 1930 the *Evening News* agonised over the plight of the Anglo-Chinese 'half-castes' of London's East End: 'the boys find work hard to get, and the girls drift about the streets ostracised by white girls of their own age. They, and not the white wives, are the broken blossoms' (quoted in Seed 2006: 67).

Novelists also reflected the 'tragedy' of these children; in Keate Weston's 1934 novel *London Fog*,[6] about a Tanganyikan student studying in London, his friendship with a white waitress leads a policewoman to warn her:

> 'Black and white mustn't mix, my dear. Not in that way. I have seen a good deal of it down at the docks, and believe me, it always ends in tragedy for both. And then – think of the children!'
>
> (quoted in Banton 1995: 195)

Such attitudes were given credence by the work of social scientists who, heavily influenced by the eugenicist tradition, were at the vanguard of a stream of investigations into this and other issues resulting from the country's 'colour problem' (Rich 1990; Bland 2005, 2007). Most notorious is Muriel Fletcher's 1930 study into the welfare of 'half-castes': *Report on an Investigation into the Colour Problem in Liverpool and Other Ports*. In response to the findings of Rachel Fleming, an anthropologist who had studied racial 'hybrids' in Britain and abroad, the Liverpool Association for the Welfare of Half-Caste Children was founded to conduct research into this 'serious problem' and Fletcher was commissioned to undertake the investigation (Rich 1990; Bland 2007; Christian 2008).

Fletcher's report was damning. In addition to its salacious and judgemental commentary about the relationships between black men and white women in particular, it concluded that the offspring of such alliances not only suffered from inherent physical and mental defects and an antipathy to work but were also socially outcast. Therefore, she concluded:

> The children find their lives full of conflict both within themselves and within the family, and all the circumstances of their lives tend to give undue prominence to sex. These families have a low standard of life, morally and economically, and there appears to be little future for the children.
>
> (quoted in Christian 2008: 230)

As Christian (2008) so expertly illustrates, although the report written by Fletcher was both methodologically flawed and heavily condemned by the local community, overall it was not only well received but profoundly influential, both at the time and in the years to come. The Fletcher report was followed by a slew of similar social scientific investigations and studies which highlighted the extent and presence of 'the colour problem' in British cities, including that of racial mixing. Though some were more sympathetic to the social and economic conditions in which these individuals, couples and families found themselves (e.g. Sharpe 1934; Hare 1937; Caradog Jones 1940), the majority continued to reinforce the overriding theme of Fletcher's work: that racial mixing was not something that 'respectable' women did and that – particularly when conducted between black men and white women – it resulted in a marginal, if not deplorable, state for all parties.[7]

With popular social objections and concerns about racial mixing now propped up by research, the undesirability of racial mixing and mixedness became firmly entrenched as common 'fact'. Thus, though the return to full employment and the more general over-riding demands of the Second World War appears to have modified intergroup hostility and improved racial attitudes in Britain thoughout the 1940s (Banton 1953), official concerns about racial mixing and 'miscegenation' were still steadfastly in place.

The reluctantly agreed presence of 'coloured' troops from the Commonwealth and USA brought this issue to the forefront of institutional interest once more. In particular, the arrival of black American GIs in 1942 caused endless consternation for British officials who were concerned about upsetting relations in the colonies if they formally supported American segregation practices. Yet, not to do so also suggested the likelihood of interracial relationships and 'half-caste babies' which some felt would have a negative effect both on the morale of white British soldiers abroad as well as on the boundaries of British national and racial identity itself (Smith 1987; Schaffer 2006; Wynn 2006).

This perplexing issue led to an on-going debate between ministers and MPs who desperately sought solutions to prevent British 'stock' being contaminated without appearing to support segregation (Smith 1987; Schaffer 2006; Wynn 2006) including, Schaffer (2006: 407–8) notes, stationing black troops in Europe – 'to fertilise the Italians who are used to it anyhow' – and introducing anti-miscegenation legislation. The rejection of the latter, Schaffer argues (2006: 408), was due more to the British reluctance to implode the country's liberal self-image by enshrining racial issues in law (and the subsequent implications of this for colonial relations), than institutional acceptance of racial mixing.

Certainly, the lack of legislation did not mean lack of condemnation; though they may not have been as explicit as the Americans, the British authorities also discouraged relationships between white British women and black – and other minority ethnic – troops in a number of ways. In addition to attempts to isolate black soldiers from the white female population through social segregation at dance halls, pubs and cinemas (Rose 1997; Wynn 2006), as Reynolds (1985: 127) notes, 'intensive efforts' were made to control women's behaviour. Female military personnel fraternising with black troops were subject to be transferred and the Auxiliary Territorial Service[8] tried to forbid its members to 'speak with coloured American soldiers except in the presence of a white [person]'.

To deal with civilians, social disapproval was the British method of control with military authorities resorting to 'covert operations', such as encouraging 'well-to-do ladies' to start whispering campaigns about venereal disease and black men, as well as the appropriate conduct for white women (Reynolds 1985; Smith 1987; Toole 1993). Moreover, in some communities, young women who were seen out with black Americans were put under surveillance and frequently monitored by specifically hired women police officers. Some women were apprehended and prosecuted under charges of loitering or trespassing, with such police action detailed in local newspapers to act as a further deterrent (Reynolds 1985; Smith 1987; Rose 1997).

These actions did little, however, to stop these interracial relationships and the inevitable presence of children born to black American soldiers caused another level of official consternation.[9] Though estimates of this group have been placed at around 1,000–1,700, far lower than the estimates of the 20,000 or so children fathered by white GIs (Reynolds 1985; Baker 1996), there was considerable debate about the 'brown baby problem', the majority of whom were illegitimate.[10] Although a few marriages to black GIs did take place (Wynn 2006), these were complicated by the fact that interracial marriage was illegal in many American states – white women relocating there, as Smith illustrates, could be jailed and deported (Smith 1987).

A widely canvassed solution, particularly amongst black American and black British community leaders, was for the children to be shipped to the US and to live with their fathers or be adopted by black families. Due to legal concerns as well as the effect transporting 'brown babies' would have on colonial relations this idea, however, was eventually dropped. So the majority of the children remained in Britain, many in state care where 'their colour made adoption unlikely' (Smith 1987: 211–13). Despite their status as British subjects, these children 'were not imagined as present or future citizens but as "problems" that should be exported' (Carby 2009: 650).

The suggestion to 'export' populations was a typical reaction to racial 'problems' on the part of British officials,[11] and in the case of Chinese sailors based in Britain during the Second World War, they were much more successful. In the early 1940s, an estimated 20,000 Chinese merchant sailors were recruited into the British Merchant Navy and, almost entirely based in Liverpool, around 300 of these married or cohabitated with local women. Although the Chinese sailors played a vital role in Britain's warfare, their demands for the same pay and equal treatment as local sailors in 1942, which led to strike action, saw them labelled as troublemakers. Post-war, the government, in collusion with the shipping companies, were keen to rid Liverpool of what they saw as an 'undesirable element' and in 1945 they were made to take one-way voyages back to China. With many blacklisted by the shipping companies, return to Britain was impossible. As has been identified through recently released records, those who had families were not given an opportunity to stay, as the law prescribed. More than 200 were suddenly and forcefully repatriated, leaving behind distraught families who believed themselves abandoned.[12]

Foley notes that though records indicate over 300 women and approximately 1,000 children were left destitute, little concern was given to the families left behind – the women were dismissively referred to in Home Office records as 'belonging to the "prostitute class"',[13] a pervasive stereotype regarding women who crossed racial boundaries. The moral outrage and panic frequently whipped up by officialdom and the media at the crossing of racial boundaries tended to be given added prurience by constantly linking it to what the *Daily Express* called the 'lowest class' of white women.[14]

Tabili (1996) expertly unravels the tangled prejudices not only towards race, but also gender and class in the imaginings of mixed-race families and people, noting that the term 'prostitute' was often used to label women – particularly working-class women – who simply diverged from prescribed norms. By transgressing racial boundaries, she argues, interracial couples also threatened to disarrange class and gender hierarchies. Their privileged middle-class – and often female – commentators denounced white working- and middle-class women who partnered men outside their race as 'unchaste' and 'bad mothers' who contributed to imperial decline as much through their deviation from class-based norms of womanly respectability as through their failure to maintain racial boundaries. Interestingly, instances of racial mixing amongst the upper classes were largely absent from social science commentary, though they did not escape social scrutiny – such as in the case of Nancy Cunard, the British aristocrat who had a high-profile affair with Henry Crowder, an African-American musician (see Joannou 2004).

Tabili makes the important point that, within this rhetoric, minority ethnic women were almost completely overlooked – though their numbers were undoubtedly small, when present they also partnered and raised families with minority men, as well as white Britons. Yet, with the exception of the pathological stereotype of the 'half-caste' girl, their presence has been even more greatly erased from historical memory, reinforcing the view that interracial relations 'were the products of a pathological attraction between white women and Black men, rather than of the more mundane desire to establish a home and family' (Tabili 1996: 183). Meanwhile, whilst for white women to risk 'polluting' the British racial stock was both degenerate and unpatriotic, the crossing of boundaries for white British men presented less of an issue; though frowned upon, it was – as during slavery – not as threatening to the racial order of Empire in which the 'preservation' of whiteness was a women's responsibility.[15]

By the 1950s, however, race had become something to tread more carefully around, at least in officialdom. After the War and the horror of the Holocaust, eugenic thinking became increasingly discredited, along with the idea that race was a biological, rather than social construction; in 1951, UNESCO's Statement on Race declared, 'there is no evidence for the existence of so-called "pure" races [and] no biological justification exists for prohibiting inter-marriage between persons of different races' (UNESCO 1969).

Yet, though racial mixing and mixedness would not be so routinely condemned by officials and institutions in the vituperative tones of the earlier half of the century, the effects would linger. Post-war, the combination of economic gloom with a visible minority ethnic presence would, once more, see the resurgence of prejudice, blame and pathologisation of minority ethnic people, including those mixing or of mixed race. Assumptions about this group were now deeply rooted in the British social psyche and it would not be until the late 1980s/early 1990s – when a 'new wave' of social science research on mixedness emerged – that perceptions about this group would begin to be deeply challenged (Caballero 2005).

Faced with such attitudes, these accounts paint a grim picture of life for mixed-race couples and people in early–mid twentieth-century Britain. Yet the frequency of what appear to be such clear social transgressions can't help but raise a question mark about the actual everyday experience of racial mixing during this time. As Bland (2005: 52) rightly notes, what is still missing in the story of those mixing and of mixed race 'in the face of a barrage of both official and cultural hostility' are the accounts of the people themselves. The next section attempts to help redress this, by highlighting in particular the voices of those who experienced and lived 'mixedness' first hand.

The 'ordinariness' of mixing and mixedness

As we have seen, the picture of racial mixing and mixedness in the first half of the twentieth century as created by the media, officials and other authorities is one that is firmly rooted in what might be called the prevailing orthodoxy of the interracial experience: marginality, conflict, rejection and confusion. It is also one in which the voices of those individuals who have experienced mixedness first hand are noticeably overlooked. Nevertheless, though uncovering these presents the well-known difficulties of unearthing the experiences of minority ethnic peoples in British history generally (Bressey 2002) – such voices are undoubtedly present.

Moreover, when we look beyond official narratives to these personal accounts, a much more complex, even contrary, picture of mixing and mixedness can be glimpsed. Take, for example, the portrayal of mixed-race children in Canning Town in the interwar period as described in this *Daily Express* article:

> There are about 600 children in all and in 98 per cent of cases their mother is white. Poor little half-castes, looked down and jeered at from their childhood upwards. … Born in a strange, murky, hostile land, brought up amid sneers and insults, launched while still in their teens upon a life barren of

> almost everything but dirt, disease and despair, without race, with no country that they can call their own, knowing no tongue but the cockney idiom of their tormentors, outcast and bereft of friends … these are the little Londoners whom human mercy and kindness seem to have passed by.[16]

Yet the identification of accounts from those who were themselves mixing and of mixed race in East London during this time period reveals perspectives that directly challenge this representation. Stephen Bourne's interviews with Anita and Christopher Crozier, the children of a Guyanese father and a white English mother who grew up in East London in the 1930s, give the impression of living in a community in which mixed families and people were not only visible but accepted:

> So black men married white women and quite a lot of mixed marriages turned out alright because they were good to each other. Where we lived there was no feeling that mixed marriages were wrong. The white people we lived with accepted it. I feel there is more racism here now than we ever had before the war. We never had any racism when I was young.
>
> (Anita Crozier, quoted in Bourne 2001: 39)

This view is also echoed in accounts of white residents, such as Doris, who also remembers growing up alongside black and mixed families in Canning Town during the same time with little racial tension in the community:

> There were lots of black kids. We used to play together, no animosity between any of us. There were white women married black, you know, West Indians, they were working on the boats. Got on ever so well together. … Everybody in the street used to speak to each other, and all the children used to play together. Sometimes when me and my sister's talking, we say, 'I wonder what happened to so and so,' you know. During the war a lot of them went.
>
> (quoted in Padfield 1999: 103)

This type of familiar, unremarkable account highlights not only the existence of this group in early twentieth-century Britain, but a sense of them living everyday lives, despite the overarching sense of official social condemnation directed at them. A glimpse at portrait and family photographs of mixed-race people, couples and families further reinforces this idea of normalcy. In their showcasing of typical family groupings or special occasions, such photographs contrast starkly with official depictions which seemed to suggest those mixing and of mixed race were so abnormal that the everyday workings and concerns of life were far beyond their scope (see the Appendix at the end of this chapter).

Indeed, in a similar vein to the work of Weeks *et al.* (2001) on sexuality in twentieth-century Britain, throughout the personal accounts of mixed-race people, families and couples runs very much a notion of the 'ordinary' – that is, 'ordinary people and ordinary lives made extraordinary by the circumstances in which they find themselves' (Weeks *et al.* 2001: preface). Certainly, many of these people, couples and families faced extraordinary levels of racism directed towards them, not only that which condemned and stigmatised them socially, but that which manifested through policy and practice. Yet for the most part, our understandings of these experiences of mixedness have been shaped by the observations or recounting of 'outsiders' whose middle-class notions of respectability and morality shaped the dominant narrative. Very rarely do we hear how such racism and prejudice affected mixed-race people, couples and families from their own perspective. Nevertheless, when such voices are heard, these take on a dimension of emotion and intimacy absent from outsider accounts. Nora, the daughter of a Monrovian father and a Welsh mother, was born in Butetown, Cardiff in 1925. Her memories of the discrimination faced by many young mixed-race women seeking employment in the 1930s highlight the depersonalisation in the findings of such studies as Muriel Fletcher's, which spoke of 'half-caste' girls 'disinclined to work':

> Well, we had terrible factories and young coloured girls or black girls, whichever they prefer to be called, had hard times finding work. … You couldn't go and work in a shop or work in an office. You had to either work in the paper works or Sigmunds or one of them paper bag factories or potato factory, anything that was nasty and grubby, you could work at. … A lot of people died before and around the war with TB from nasty places. Lots of very beautiful half-caste and black children died from working in these menial places during the war because the places were damp and dirty and that was the only way we could work.[17]

The prevalence of outsider views has also meant that the ways in which such prejudiced practices and portrayals were refuted and challenged by the individuals and families themselves are overlooked. Certainly, during those periods when public condemnation of racial mixing and mixedness was virulent, can be found evidence of resistance – powerful and subtle – by mixed-race people and families themselves. Christian (2008: 222) reports that Fletcher was 'stabbed and run out of the city' by outraged locals after the publication of her report and Kenneth Little (1972: 134) notes in his 1940s research on Butetown:

> the term 'Half-Caste' is the name in general use by the outsider. It is as well to note, however, that it is rarely if ever used within the community, and is very unpopular among the young people concerned, who usually prefer to be referred to as 'coloured.'

Such protests and objections, however, were rarely given voice outside the communities, though occasionally they did reach wider audiences, such as through rebuttals in the letters pages of local and national papers:

> As for the coloured men being inferior, well, it may be only in stature, but they are kind and gentle to their wives and children and that is more than a great deal of the so-called white men can say. Even if the coloured gentlemen of Holborn [district in South Shields] had to resort to sell

> oranges they would do it willingly to support the white wife they chose to share their lives and their kiddies; they look after their own and take care of what they have.
>
> 'A White Woman of Six'[18]

Similar types of letter, mostly written by white women, can be found in other local and national newspapers, with many referring to the happiness and harmony present in interracial family life. In a number of ways, it would seem that the unity of the family was a key means of resistance and support against the pernicious racism and prejudice directed towards those who were in or from mixed-race relationships. 'Marital' satisfaction was also commented upon by social scientists who, sometimes in surprised tones, noted high levels of affection and harmony displayed in interracial families, not only between husband and wives, but between the parents and the children. In addition, the critical role of white wives in fighting for and accessing resources, such as jobs or housing, for their husbands is also often noted (e.g. Hare 1937; Richmond 1954; Collins 1957; Little 1972).

Furthermore, though certainly many white women who partnered men from other cultures in the inter and post-war years were shunned by their extended families, these family units were not automatically marginalised from extended family networks. Tabili's (1996: 181) claim that in seaport communities, interracial couples could be found 'living in the same house with the wives' families, a common working-class residential pattern' is confirmed by other mid-twentieth-century studies of these communities (e.g. Richmond 1954; Collins 1957; Little 1972).

Similarly, despite the prevailing social condemnation, public attitudes towards mixed-race people, couples and families were not always antagonistic. The friendliness of white Britons towards black GIs, for example, at least during the early years of the Second World War, has been well documented (e.g. Smith 1987; Gough 2007). Nava (2007: 76) convincingly argues that the outcome of a 1943 Mass-Observation survey which showed 'one in seven disapprove of mixed marriages' does not support the contention of 'near-universal hostility towards interracial sexual relations' that has been attributed to white Britons during this time. Certainly, as Kushner (2004: 22) illustrates in his wonderful research into the Mass-Observation archives, for some, it was possible to regard racial mixing as 'an ordinary part of the local landscape'. Such was the case in 1939 for a 26-year-old white male diarist from Newport:

> I could visualise myself falling in love with a negress. If I did, I wouldn't hesitate about marrying her. … I have known a lot of cases of mixed marriages here [in Newport] and Cardiff and Barry, although they have all been cases of white women marrying black men. In fact, there is a street in Newport entirely occupied by such couples. The women seem happy and the men treat them well. My Sunday school work brought me into contact with some of the children of such marriages. They seemed very bright,

> clever people, and very happy. The attitude of the white children was interesting. They accepted the others quite naturally, even 'palled up' with them. Among these children, at any rate, there was no 'colour bar'.

Of course, we need to be careful not to essentialise these memories of 'ordinariness' so that they speak for or to the experiences of all mixed-race people and couples, or diminish those experiences of racism and prejudice of which there are undoubtedly many. Rather, we need to recognise the range of accounts and realise how such polarities can form part of the complexity and diversity of mixing and mixedness, within and across experiences. Certainly, in both official and first-hand accounts, we repeatedly see the presence of what Les Back (1996) has called the 'metropolitan paradox', the complex and fascinating intersection of multiculture and racism where, particularly in the port cities, a picture emerges of localities in which attitudes towards mixedness veered between acceptance and antipathy. Like many other Butetown residents in the 1930s and 1940s – then often referred to as 'Tiger Bay' – Nora (introduced earlier) remembers mixedness as a very ordinary part of growing up:

> I grew up as the average child in the Bay of a mixed family … And I lived in Loudon Square which had 62 houses and about 42 nations in each. … People were really lovely, they were nice people, very human, very nice. They had their ups, their downs, … they were just hardworking mixed families, most of whom were very well respected. Very few of them ever got into trouble and went to jail out of the old times. It was just a happy life, with all nations of the world.

However, whilst this mixedness might have been an ordinary part of Butetown life, Nora recalls that things were different in central Cardiff where racial mixing was 'resented' and where, consequently, many couples did not venture:

> Most of the fathers went uptown, but a lot of the mothers never went uptown, we shopped and bought everything in The Bay … and mothers and fathers didn't go over the bridge very often, because they were abused.

Such polarities could also be found outside the city. As today, mixed racial and ethnic relationships and people were not simply a preserve of city life (Caballero *et al.* 2008). Indeed, there are fascinating glimpses of mixing and mixedness to be found in the suburbs, towns and rural communities of Britain even before the twentieth century (e.g. MacKeith 2003; Livesay 2010). Alfred Lawes, who grew up in the 1930s in Maerdy, a mining village in rural Wales, was the son of a West Indian father and a Welsh mother. He talks about growing up as part of a tight-knit community where his father, who had come looking for work in the mines with other former black sailors, had met and married his mother:

> They were accepted. My father was black, my mother was white. But that was it. They accepted them and of course as we came along, my brother and my sister as well, we were accepted as one … And I can honestly say

> this. That although down in Butetown, Cardiff, they weren't allowed out of it very much, in Maerdy they were part of it, they were exactly the same as if they were born in Maerdy.[19]

For Alfred, it was only when he left Maerdy that his race became an issue, when he was prevented from serving in India during the Second World War ('I was the wrong colour to go to India. And that was the first time [I had experienced prejudice], you see'), thus highlighting once again the multifaceted and shifting nature of the mixed experience. Though we still know little about the history of the rural and suburban minority ethnic presence in Britain, accounts of black soldiers during the Second World War,[20] who were mostly stationed in small towns of England, indicate that, as in the cities, acceptance and antagonism were both often present in the mixed experience. As a relative of Joan Artis, a white woman who married Jack, a black British soldier, in Kent recalls:

> They were married [in 1944] for fifty plus years until [Jack's] death in 1997 ... He told us that the worst racism he came across was from white American GIs. ... My aunt summed this up with a story of the family meeting up at the local pub when a leave allowed them to virtually all be together, that is all the uncles who were serving, plus the aunts and grandpa. Into the pub came some white GIs, apparently some snide remarks were not long forthcoming from the GIs all aimed at Uncle Jack. The GIs, however, got more than they bargained for as the people in the pub (besides our family) all knew and liked Jack well. The GIs were turned upon and after a 'scuffle' were unceremoniously ejected from the pub and told not to return again in no uncertain terms.[21]

Looking at these accounts, what becomes clear is the oscillating nature of the mixed experience where the shift from 'fitting in' to 'standing out' depending on the circumstances of locality can be abrupt and sudden. Yet, of course, geography is not alone in shaping this – gender, class, economic status, local and national politics amongst other factors intersect to make racial mixing and mixedness a complex and diverse experience, sometimes shared, sometimes unique. Though often connected by the shared thread of discrimination and prejudice, the experiences of mixing or mixedness amongst the upper classes in the mid-twentieth century, such as those of Nancy Cunard and Henry Crowder or Noor Inayat Khan,[22] often differ greatly from each other as well as from those in dockland communities. Through uncovering their voices, however, the possibility of understanding the complexity and diversity of their experience becomes stronger.

Conclusion

For those mixing and of mixed race in Britain in the period between 1920 and 1950, it is clear that they did so against a social discourse and set of attitudes which, particularly at an official, institutional level, positioned them as unnatural, unsettling and unwanted. For many, this social condemnation had painful or brutal consequences: interracial couples being attacked or torn apart, those from mixed-race backgrounds being refused work and opportunities, mixed-race children shipped off to orphanages to avoid social disgrace and all against a discursive backdrop which labelled such families and peoples as immoral, feckless, degenerate and dangerous.

Yet, amongst all the moral condemnation, there is nevertheless a sense of ordinariness. The concept of 'ordinary' may seem unusual when applied to racial mixing and its familiar setting of ostracism, marginalisation, 'tragic mulattoes' and 'marginal men'. Nevertheless, it is there, in both the extent of its presence and its matter-of-factness, the negotiation of those social and practical issues, big and small, which people faced on an everyday level, regardless of their race or colour: friendship, love, marriage, children, money, work, death, cleaning, cooking, decorating, shopping, socialising, parenting.

As Green (2000) has pointed out, understandings of the history of minority ethnic peoples in Britain are often restricted by assumptions about both the longevity of their presence and their diverse and multifaceted nature. Such it is with racially mixed people, couples and families. In this respect, reclaiming the 'ordinariness' of their history is extremely important. With the history of racial mixing and mixedness having long been presented to us largely through, as Balachandran (2011: 27–28) notes, the 'prurient gaze of middle-class observers peering through lens clouded by class, racial, gender, sexual and political anxieties', it is now timely to develop 'new narratives through which everyday experience is being reordered and new meanings emerge' (Weeks *et al.* 2001: 6). Though there is much more work to be done in uncovering these new narratives – particularly in collecting more contextually detailed reminiscences – the inclusion of personal accounts certainly allows us to highlight a more complex picture of mixing and mixedness than has traditionally been painted.

The importance of a more multidimensional history of mixedness is also critical for informing contemporary experiences. Certainly, prevailing official and social attitudes to mixing and mixedness have changed dramatically from the time of 'Draughtboard Alley'. Yet though 'Brown Britain' is more likely to be heralded as 'Britain's beautiful future' than its problem, racism – both explicit and institutional – still continues to inform and affect the lives of mixed-race people and families.[23] Often this is expressed through traditional pathologisations which see mixed-race children as inherently 'marooned between communities' and their parents as of dubious sexual morals (Caballero 2010). Yet, once more, such patterns and assumptions aren't always borne out in contemporary accounts or are the sum and total of the experience of mixed-race people and their families. Indeed, contemporary accounts also indicate an overlooked sense of 'ordinariness', where many of those difficulties and challenges pointed to those mixing and of mixed race relate to wider social attitudes rather than their own internal contradictions, confusions or culture clashes (e.g. Tikly *et al.* 2004; Caballero *et al.* 2008).

As accounts of mixedness from earlier in the twentieth century start to be uncovered, it's important to acknowledge the diversity – both of situation and experience – that lies within them, particularly the recognition that though we may discover some patterns in common, we can't necessarily assume these will be the case for everyone. Undoubtedly, the diversity and complexity of the lives of those mixing and of mixed-race backgrounds is so much deeper than can be explained by the casual generalisations and assumptions that have defined their history so far. The 'ordinary' stories of 'everyday' people of mixed race – both now and then – are seldom told, but they are critical in presenting a more balanced picture of the experiences of 'mixedness' – one that is not all about cultural harmony and acceptance but equally one that is not all about tragedy, prejudice and difficulty. For when we slowly begin to uncover such accounts, which include the good, the bad and the quite simply mundane, we can start to see this generally hidden history of racial mixing in Britain as simply another part of the longstanding diversity and difference that is – and always has been – an ordinary feature of British life.

Appendix

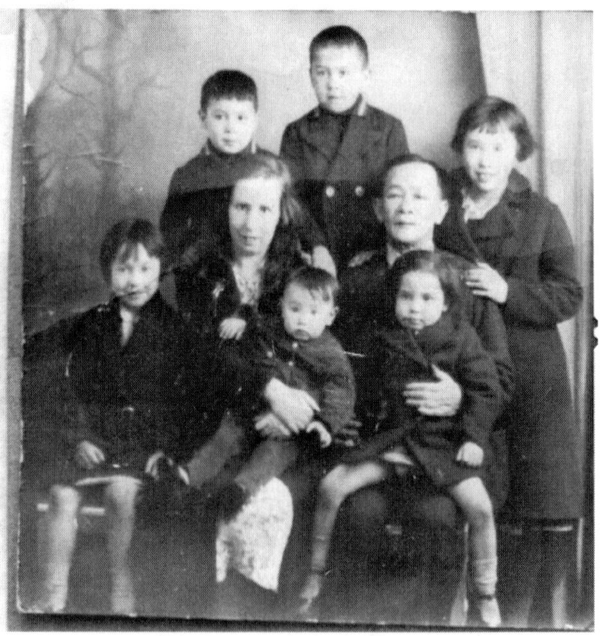

Figure 4.1 Unknown Anglo-Chinese family, Liverpool, *c*.1930s. Courtesy of Yvonne Foley

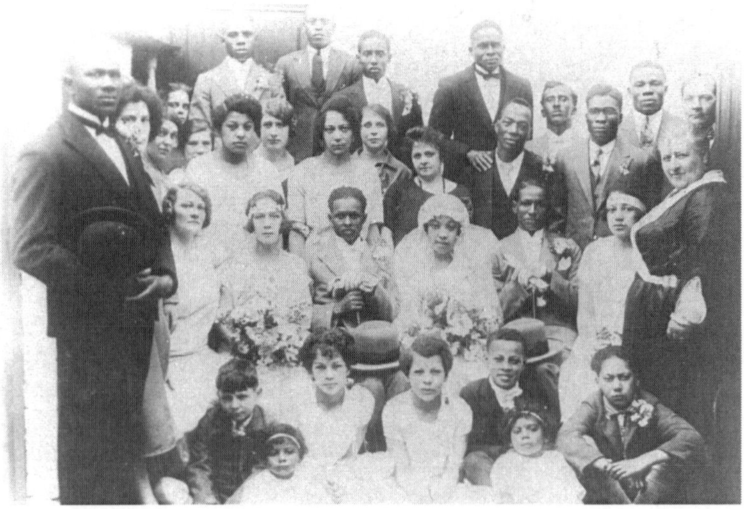

Figure 4.2 Wedding party of Mohammed Hassan, Somali, and Katie Link, mixed-race Welsh, in Butetown, *c.*1925. Courtesy of Butetown History and Arts Centre

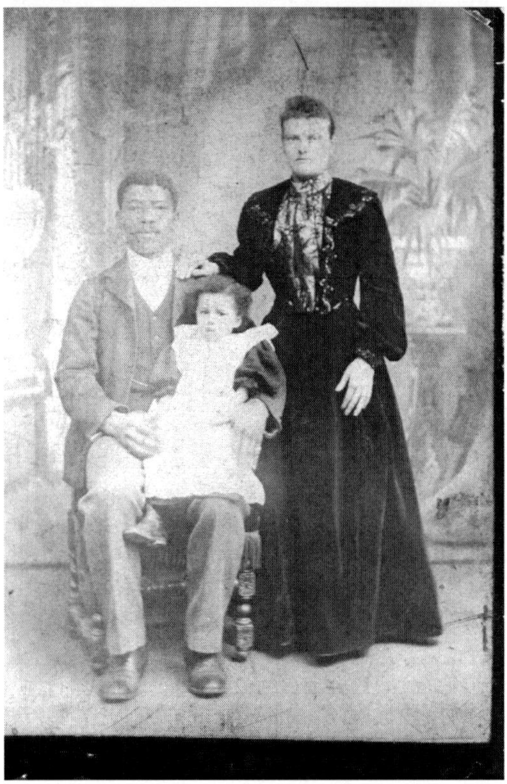

Figure 4.3 Unknown family portrait, *c.*1916. Courtesy of Butetown Archives and Heritage Centre

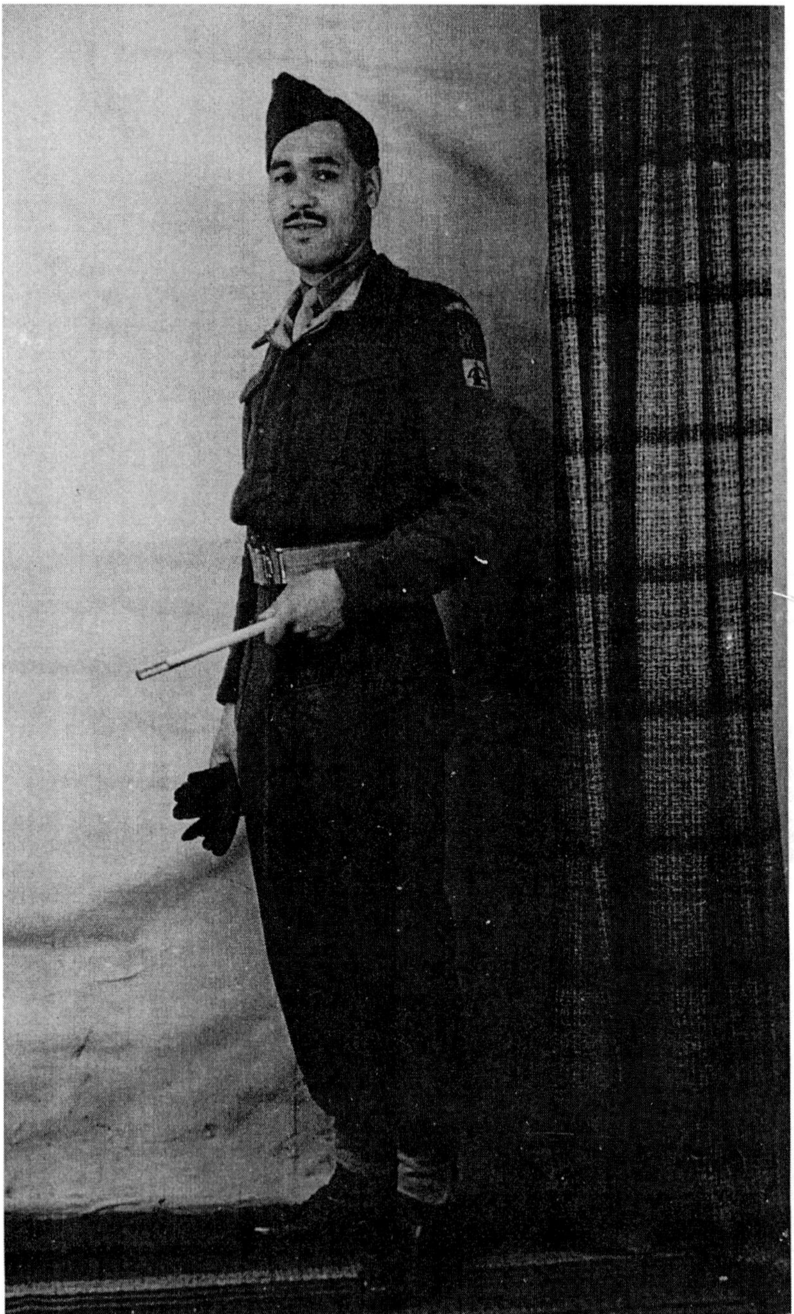

Figure 4.4 Reuben St Claire, platoon officer in the Home Guard, son of Joseph, a black Barbadian dentist and Mabel, a white Bristolian, *c.*1940–45. Courtesy of Bristol Record Office

Notes

1 With thanks to Peter Aspinall for his invaluable comments and input.
2 The *Guardian*, 22 May 1997; *Mail on Sunday*, 8 December 2002.
3 'The era of moral condemnation: mixed race people in Britain, 1920–50', Chamion Caballero (London South Bank University) and Peter Aspinall (University of Kent), 2007. This project was funded by The British Academy (Ref: SG-47233).
4 See later in the chapter for discussion of minority ethnic women and racial mixing in Britain.
5 The 1914 British Nationality and Status of Aliens Act – which saw British women who married 'aliens' lose 'the rights and privileges accorded to British nationality' – was not reformed until 1948. See Baldwin (2001).
6 With thanks to Michael Banton for highlighting the representation of black men in London in novels of the early 1930s.
7 See, for example, Captain F.A. Richardson's 1935 report on *Social Conditions in Ports and Dockland Areas*; the Rev. St John Groser *et al.*'s 1942 report on *Conditions of Life of the Coloured Population of Stepney*; Mrs Phyllis Young's 1944 *Report on an Investigation into the Conditions of the Coloured Population in a Stepney area* (see Banton 1953, 1955; Little 1972; Tabili 1996).
8 The women's branch of the British Army during the war.
9 Interestingly, there seems to have been little official focus on children born to fathers of other ethnic minorities during wartime, possibly because, as Rose (1997: 155) suggests, such children were mostly seen as a problem 'hidden' in working-class port communities, rather than the nationwide issue the 'brown babies' became.
10 White American officers invariably refused permission for black soldiers to marry their white girlfriends.
11 As after the 1919 riots when voluntary repatriation was made available to all 'coloured' colonial soldiers (Bland 2005; Tabili 1994).
12 Yvonne Foley, http://www.halfandhalf.org.uk/index and http://www.movinghere.org.uk/stories/Story581/Story581.htm?identifier=stories/Story581/Story581.htm, accessed 24 April 2011. Also *The Shanghai Sailors*, BBC Radio 4, broadcast 13 September 2008.
13 Yvonne Foley, http://www.halfandhalf.org.uk/index, accessed 24 April 2011.
14 *Daily Express*, 18 June 1923.
15 Bland (2005) notes that although the 1903 Immorality Suppression Ordinance in the British colony of Southern Rhodesia outlawed sex outside marriage between white women and black men, no such legislation prohibited sex between white men and black women until 1927 and, even then, such transgressions were perceived as a far lesser crime.
16 *Daily Express*, 18 March 1930.
17 Interview with Nora Glasgow, Butetown Community History Project.
18 *Shields Daily Gazette*, 23 March 1923 (in Lawless 1995: 185–86).
19 Source: Millennium Memory Bank.
20 For more on local and national attitudes to black GIs and colonial soldiers and workers see, for example, Richmond 1954, Smith 1987 and Wynn, 2006.
21 'My Black Uncle, WW2 People's War', http://www.bbc.co.uk/ww2peopleswar, accessed 3 January 2012.
22 The British-born daughter of an Indian Muslim Prince and a white American mother who worked as a Special Operations Executive agent in the Second World War.
23 The *Guardian*, 15 August 2011.

References

Ansari, H. (2004) *The Infidel Within: Muslims in Britain since 1800*, London: Hurst & Company.

Back, L. (1996) *New Ethnicities and Urban Culture: Racisms and Multiculture in Young Lives*, Oxford: Routledge.

Baker, J. (1996) 'The Children They Left Behind', *Lest We Forget* 4(2). http://www.coax.net/people/lwf/CHILDREN.HTM, accessed 14 October 2010.

Balachandran, G. (2011) 'Subaltern Cosmopolitanism in the Imperial Metropole: Notes Towards a Prehistory of Racism and Multiculturalism' in *Working Papers in International History*, No. 8. http://graduateinstitute.ch/webdav/site/international_$history_politics/shared/working_papers/WPIHP_8_Balachandran.pdf, accessed 3 January 2012.

Baldwin, M.P. (2001) 'Subject to Empire: Married Women and the British Nationality and Status of Aliens Act' in *Journal of British Studies*, 40: 522–56.

Banton, M. (1953) 'The Changing Position of the Negro in Britain' in *Phylon*, 14(1): 74–83.

——(1955) *The Coloured Quarter: Negro Immigrants in an English City*, London: Jonathan Cape.

——(1995) 'The Black Man in London in the Early 1930s: A Note on Some Novels' in *Immigrants and Minorities*, 14(2): 195–99.

BBC (n.d.) 'My Black Uncle, WW2 People's War', http://www.bbc.co.uk/ww2peopleswar, accessed 3 January 2012.

BBC Radio 4, *The Shanghai Sailors*, broadcast 13 September 2008.

Bland, L. (2005) 'White Women and Men of Colour: Miscegenation Fears in Britain After the Great War' in *Gender and History*, 17(1): 29–61.

——(2007) 'British Eugenics and "Race Crossing": A Study of an Interwar Investigation' in *New Formations*, 60: 66–78.

Bourne, S. (2001) *Black in the British Frame: The Black Experience in British Film and Television*, London: Continuum.

Bressey, C. (2002) 'Forgotten Histories: Three Stories of Black Girls from Barnardo's Victorian Archive' in *Women's History Review*, 11(3): 351–74.

Caballero, C. (2005) '"Mixed Race Projects": Perceptions, Constructions and Implications of Mixed Race in the UK and USA', unpublished PhD thesis, University of Bristol.

——(2010) *Lone Mothers of Mixed Racial and Ethnic Children: A Case Study*, published online by Single Parent Action Network (SPAN), http://www.one space.org.uk/your-roots/lone-mothers-mixed-race-children, accessed 3 January 2012.

Caballero, C., Edwards, R. and Puthussery, S. (2008) *Parenting 'Mixed' Children: Negotiating Difference and Belonging, in Mixed Race, Ethinicity and Faith Families*, London: Joseph Rowntree Foundation.

Caradog Jones, C. (1940) *The Economic Status of Coloured Children in the Port of Liverpool*, Liverpool: Liverpool University Press.

Carby, H. (2009) 'Becoming Modern Racialized Subjects' in *Cultural Studies*, 23(4): 624–27.

Christian, M. (2008) 'The Fletcher Report 1930: A Historical Case Study of Contested Black Mixed Heritage Britishness' in *Journal of Historical Sociology*, 21(2–3): 213–41.

Collins, S. (1957) *Coloured Minorities in Britain: Studies in British Race Relations Based on African, West Indian and Asiatic Immigration*, London: Butterworth.

Dikötter, F. (1998) 'Race Culture: Recent Perspectives on the History of Eugenics' in *The American Historical Review*, 103(2): 467–78.

Foley, Y. (n.d.) *Half and Half*, http://www.halfandhalf.org.uk/index, accessed 24 April 2011.

Foley, Y. (n.d.) *Moving Here*, http://www.movinghere.org.uk/stories/Story581/Story581.htm?identifier=stories/Story581/Story581.htm, accessed 24 April 2011.

Fryer, P. (1984) *Staying Power: The History of Black People in Britain*, London: Pluto Press.

Gough, A. (2007) 'Messing Up Another Country's Customs: The Exportation of American Racism During World War II' in *World History Connected*, www.worldhistoryconnected.press.illinois.edu/5.1/gough.html, accessed 15 April 2011.

Green, J. (2000) 'Before the Windrush' in *History Today*, 50: 29–35.

Hall, R. (1977) *Marie Stopes: A Biography*, London: André Deutsch Limited.

Hare, N. (1937) 'The Prospects for Coloured Children in England' in *The Keys*, 5(1): 11–12 and 25–27.

Joannou, M. (2004) 'Nancy Cunard's English Journey' in *Feminist Review*, 78: 141–63.

Kushner, T. (2004) *We Europeans? Mass-Observation, 'Race' and British Identity in the Twentieth Century*, Farnham: Ashgate Publishing Limited.

Lawless, R. (1995) *From Ta'izz to Tyneside: An Arab Community in the North-East of England During the Early Twentieth Century*, Exeter: University of Exeter Press.

Little, K. (1972 [1948]) *Negroes in Britain*, London: Routledge. Second edition.

Livesay, D. (2010) *Children of Uncertain Fortune: Mixed-Race Migrants from the West Indies to Britain, 1750–1820*, unpublished PhD thesis, University of Michigan.

Lorimer, D. (1978) *Colour, Class and the Victorians: English Attitudes to the Negro in the Mid-Nineteenth Century*, Leicester: Leicester University Press.

MacKeith, L. (2003) *Local Black History: A Beginning in Devon*, London: Archives and Museum of Black Heritage.

Mazumdar, P. (1991) *Eugenics, Human Genetics and Human Failings: The Eugenics Society, Its Sources and Its Critics in Britain*, London: Routledge.

Nava, M. (2007) *Visceral Cosmopolitanism: Gender, Culture and the Normalisation of Difference*, Oxford: Berg.

Padfield, D. (1999) *Hidden Lives: Stories from the East End by the People of 42 Balaam Street*, London: Eastside Community Heritage.

Reynolds, D. (1985) 'The Churchill Government and the Black American Troops in Britain During World War II' in *Transactions of the Royal Historical Society*, 35: 113–33.

Rich, P. (1990) *Race and Empire in British Politics*, Cambridge: Cambridge University Press. Second edition.

Richmond, A. (1954) *Colour Prejudice in Britain: A Study of West Indian Workers in Liverpool, 1941–1951*, London: Routledge & Kegan Paul Ltd.

Rose, S. (1997) 'Girls and GIs: Race, Sex and Diplomacy in Second World War Britain' in *The International History Review*, 19(1): 146–60.

Schaffer, G. (2006) 'Re-Thinking the History of Blame: Britain and Minorities During the Second World War' in *National Identities*, 8(4): 401–19.

Seed, J. (2006) 'Limehouse Blues: Looking for Chinatown in the London Docks, 1900–1940' in *History Workshop Journal*, 62: 58–85.

Sharpe, N. (1934) 'Cardiff's Coloured Population' in *The Keys*, 1(3): 44–45 and 61.

Smith, G. (1987) *When Jim Crow Met John Bull: Black American Soldiers in World War II Britain*, London: I.B. Tauris & Co.

Tabili, L. (1994) *'We Ask For British Justice': Workers and Racial Difference in Late Imperial Britain*, Ithaca, NY: Cornell University Press.

——(1996) '"Women of a Very Low Type": Crossing Racial Boundaries in Imperial Britain' in Frader, L. and Rose, S. (eds) *Gender and Class in Modern Europe*, Ithaca, NY: Cornell University Press, pp.165–90.

Tikly, L., Caballero, C., Haynes, J. and Hill, J. (2004) *Understanding the Educational Needs of Mixed Heritage Pupils*, London: DfES.

Toole, J. (1993) 'GIs and the Race Bar in Wartime Warrington' in *History Today*, 43(7): 23–28.

UNESCO (1969) *Four Statements on the Race Question*, Paris: UNESCO. http://unesdoc.unesco.org/images/0012/001229/122962eo.pdf, accessed 13 March 2012.

Weeks, J., Heaphy, B. and Donovan, C. (2001) *Same Sex Intimacies: Families of Choice and Other Life Experiments*, London: Routledge.

Worth, J. (2002) *Call the Midwife: A True Story of the East End in the 1950s*, London: Weidenfeld & Nicolson.

Wynn, N. (2006) '"Race War": Black American GIs and West Indians in Britain During the Second World War' in *Immigrants & Minorities*, 24(3): 324–46.

5 When ethnicity became an important family issue

The case of Slovenian Istria

Mateja Sedmak

Introduction

There has been a striking lack of theoretical and empirical work dedicated to ethnically mixed partnerships and families in Slovenia. The reasons for such lack of interest in this specific research area are a relatively high degree of ethnical homogeneity within the state (albeit with some regional exceptions)[1] and the prevailing political ideology of the former common state of Yugoslavia, which reduced the importance of ethnic affiliation. Eriksen (1993) terms this a case of undercommunication of ethnicity. Principles of "brotherhood and equality" were promoted within the frame of the socialist ideal of the former state in order to ensure interethnic equality, tolerance and coexistence as well as to strengthen the position of class above the attributed ethnic determinants. The paucity of research interest in relationships between partners from different ethnic backgrounds can be seen as a by-product of an ideologically conceived ideal of interethnic equality and assumptions that did not problematize the social and research components of ethnic issues. Simultaneously, however, the ideology of interethnic equality gave rise to considerable ethnic heterogamy in the territory of former Yugoslavia.

Slovenia's independence in 1991, its entry into the European Union in 2004, and the consequences of global trends such as increased spacial mobility, mass economic migration, intercultural contacts and exchanges, have provoked a growing interest in the area of ethnic issues and ethnically mixed families. Following the period of independence, members of ethnically mixed families faced a number of difficulties as they underwent an "overnight" and involuntary change of status from interstate marriages and families to international marriages and families. Prior to 1991, ethnically mixed families primarily had to cope with questions of intercultural and interlinguistic adaptations and ways to harmonize different life styles, habits and values. After 1991, the introduction of national borders burdened ethnically mixed families with new, potentially stressful situations in which they were confronted with the need to find survival strategies for altered circumstances. Within this framework, the mixed families consisting of Slovenes and members of other nationalities of former Yugoslavia were most affected.

In this chapter I draw on my research into ethnically mixed families in Slovene Istria.[2] This is a border area that, unlike other areas in Slovenia, is distinguished by a high degree of cultural, linguistic and religious diversity, and partnerships across them. In many respects, partnership and family dynamics in ethnically mixed families do not differ from ethnically homogenous families; they face similar everyday issues of interpersonal adaptation, economic supply, children's socialization, and emotional and social care for extended family members (Romano 1988). Indeed, the accounts from members of ethnically mixed families that I report on in this chapter reveal that love, mutual care and closeness are the most important issues for them. Issues arising from cultural, linguistic, racial and religious differences are secondary (Sedmak 2002a). According to Ibrahim and Schroeder (1990), partners in a mixed family need to invest additional effort because they often are confronted with conflict situations that do not arise from their character or personal nature, but rather stem from their incompatible cultural patterns. The need for partner and family self-reflection increases with greater cultural distance. But we also need to consider the importance and influence of the intolerant, xenophobic, nationalist and racist environment that I discuss below.

My contribution in this chapter focuses on the effects of intercultural contacts on the interpersonal level of everyday life, especially levels of satisfaction with life in ethnically mixed families, the response of extended family members and of children; and – last but not least – the consequences of political and social changes in the 1990s for members of ethnically mixed families. First, however, I set the scene for understanding the phenomenon of partnering across different ethnic backgrounds in Slovenia by discussing some key characteristics of interethnic relations in Slovene Istria.

Interethnic relations in Slovene Istria

The theory of spatial ethnic concentration identifies three types of area characterized by high levels of ethnic pluralism in contemporary Europe: border areas, highly industrialized and urbanized areas that are particularly attractive to economic migrants, and multinational states (Sussi 1994). The territory of Slovene Istria meets all three criteria: it is a border area lying between Italy and Croatia in the south-western part of Slovenia with access to the Adriatic Sea; there is a port – Luka Koper – and strong local industry; and it used to draw internal economic migrants from other territories of former Yugoslavia. In addition, economically Slovene Istria is the second most developed and wealthy region in the state, characterized by one of the lowest unemployment rates, and it also possesses a favourable geographic and border position and mild climate that makes it attractive to a broader circle of immigrants.

Despite a constant decrease over the last 60 years, Slovenes still account for the largest share of the population (68.3 per cent), followed by Croats (4.8 per cent), Serbs (3.4 per cent), Bosnians (3.2 per cent) and members of the Italian minority (2.3 per cent). Other ethnicities (Macedonians, Montenegrins, Albanians, etc.)

account for less than 1 per cent of the entire population. Almost certainly, however, there is a huge discrepancy between statistical data and the real situation; the number of people belonging to non-Slovene ethnicities is significantly higher. One of the obvious consequences of the spatial concentration of different ethnic groups in Slovene Istria is a relatively high number of ethnically mixed families. While the share of ethnically mixed families in Slovenia in general amounts to 20.2 per cent, in Slovene Istria it is as high as 34.8 per cent (Sedmak 2006).

Interethnic relations in Slovene Istria are influenced significantly by the presence of an Italian indigenous minority. Italians have "always" lived in the area, although over time their status has changed dramatically. Historically, Italians lived in the coastal urban centres, while Slovenes inhabited the rural hinterland of Istria, representing the lower social class; that is, the village populations. The area underwent significant demographic change after World War II. From 1918 to 1945, the territory of Slovene Istria was under Italian occupation.[3] After the end of World War II, it was first part of Zone B of Venezia Giulia and then became part of Zone B of the Free Territory of Trieste to be annexed by the Federal People's Republic of Yugoslavia after the Memorandum of London in 1954. According to this treaty, all citizens of Italian nationality were given the right to emigrate to Italy within a limited period of time (by the beginning of 1956). After the treaty, it became clear that Istria would not belong to Italy, thus triggering an exodus to Italy, primarily of citizens of Italian origin but also Slovene and Croat (Darovec 2008). Following such mass emigration and the consequent immigration of Slovenes from neighbouring villages and other Slovene regions along with inhabitants of other nationalities, the national structure of Slovene Istria changed considerably.

The citizens of Italian ethnicity who stayed were later granted official minority status and the minority rights stemming from it. The Italian minority thus is acknowledged to have the right to their mother tongue in public life and in education, as well as to cultural, economic and political organization. As a result, the Italian community is served by kindergartens, primary and secondary schools using Italian as the language of instruction; these schools are also attended by a high number of children of Slovenes and other ethnic groups. Members of the Italian community have political representatives at local and national parliamentary levels. They are characterized by a high level of cultural and social organization but by negligible economic organization, which has only been initiated in recent years (Sedmak *et al.* 2002a). Istria also has a radio and television station broadcasting in the Italian language. Moreover, bilingualism is a feature of all official documents (identity cards, passports and birth certificates), public invitations, municipal notices and so on. Attitude surveys have revealed that the local Slovene population regards members of the Italian minority as "locals", "our people" and "one of us" (Sedmak 2002a). Equally interesting, the results of linguistic research indicate a high level of Italian language competence among the majority Slovene population in Istria, with more than 90 per cent of the majority population being users of minority language (Mikolič 2003a, 2003b).

Interethnic relations in Slovene Istria are characterized by a relatively high degree of tolerance and absence of explicit expressions of nationalism or xenophobia (Sedmak *et al.* 2002b). The high level of interethnic acceptance is reinforced by the relatively high level of cross-ethnic partnering mentioned above, while the research findings also reveal that both adult and young people express a relatively high level of willingness to marry a member of another ethnic group living in the same environment (Sedmak 2003b; Sedmak *et al.* 2002b). Here, it should be emphasized that willingness to marry a member of another ethnicity demonstrates the highest level of acceptance of their members (Štrukelj 1986). Another factor that demonstrates the high level of interethnic acceptance is the enrolment of Slovene children and children of immigrant groups from the territory of former Yugoslavia in Italian-language kindergartens, primary and secondary schools. Research conducted at local Italian secondary schools in 2003 revealed that only one quarter of all students actually were members of the Italian community (Sedmak 2003b).

A full picture of the complex nature of interethnic relations in Slovene Istria needs to take into account the fact that Slovenes' attitude towards other local ethnic groups is determined by their autochthonous (indigenous) or non-autochthonous (immigrant) status. Despite being fewer in number compared to immigrant communities, members of the Italian ethnicity are granted special status and special rights stemming from their autochthonous status *per se* (Sedmak 2002a, 2003a, 2003b; Sedmak *et al.* 2002b). Furthermore, Slovenes and members of immigrant groups acknowledge (at least in principle) the justice of granting the Italian minority rights in relation to their ethnic affiliation. Regardless (or perhaps because) of a relatively low population, the Italian ethnic group is a remarkably cohesive and well-organized community with a high level of informal internal cohesion and control. The social status of the Italian minority in the local community is relatively high and so is the attendant power. The vital importance of internal cohesion and integration for the subsistence of a given (ethnic) group was underlined by Elias and Scotson (1994), who claim that this factor typically characterizes indigenous, autochthonous populations and allows a privileged position.

In contrast, while immigrants – who predominantly are from the areas of former Yugoslavia – are given political, social and economic rights according to their acquired citizenship, the Slovene state does not grant them the status of specific cultural groups, and consequently does not encourage their cultural, linguistic and religious diversity. Thus, immigrants maintain their language, culture and tradition only within their family and narrower local community.

An interesting phenomenon relating to immigrants from areas of former Yugoslavia is the non-differentiation of separate ethnicities; in the everyday perceptions and vocabulary of the Slovene and Italian populations diverse immigrant ethnicities frequently are viewed as a single immigrant group. For example, the term "Bosnian" is used by the Slovene majority to describe immigrants from former Yugoslavia who appear to have failed to integrate linguistically and culturally, regardless of their actual nationality.

The dynamics of interethnic relations seem to be embedded through intergenerational transmission of values and attitudes. There are some similarities in generational attitudes between young people and adults living in Istria (Sedmak 2003b; Sedmak *et al.* 2002b). There is a slight difference however: while the attitudes of the youth and adult populations are relatively similar in relation to the Italian autochthonous group, their attitudes towards immigrant groups and their rights differ, with significantly lower acceptance of immigrants by the young. This difference is explained by the *a priori* lower social status attached to immigrants and, importantly, by the fact that – post-independence in the 1990s – younger informants were socialized in an atmosphere of accentuated distinctions between Slovene culture on the one hand, and cultures of other nations of former Yugoslavia on the other.

The importance of autochthonous or immigrant status in everyday interethnic relations in Slovene Istria also has consequences for the life of ethnically mixed families, as I now discuss.

Intercultural confrontations at the interpersonal level of partner and family life

Thinking about intercultural encounters in family life raises issues about different cultural traditions such as ways of dressing, eating habits, values, religious practices, as well as two different languages, expectations related to sexuality, intimacy and so on (Romano 1988; Breger and Hill 1998). Which cultural elements prevail in an ethnically mixed family and why? Possible scenarios include the prevalence of one or the other culture or the coexistence or confrontation of elements of both cultures.

For mixed families living in Slovene Istria, the non-autochthonous status of a non-Slovene partner turned out to be the key challenge of intercultural confrontation in everyday life for partners and families. Thus I now consider the dualism between Slovene–Italian families (both ethnicities being autochthonous) and Slovene–ex-Yugoslavian families (marriage between members of autochthonous and immigrant ethnics) to demonstrate different perspectives of family life in mixed families.

Slovene–Italian mixed families

Birth, socialization and life in a common geographic area mean that Slovene–Italian partners consider themselves as culturally similar, except for their different languages (Sedmak 2002a). Further, the Slovene population of Istria is distinguished by a transcultural identity in which they show a higher degree of intercultural similarity to the population of neighbouring Italy than to the Slovene population from inner areas of Slovenia (Sedmak 2009). This raises the issue of the distinction between language and "the rest of the culture".

In the case of Slovene–Italian mixed marriages, there is a pattern of language pluralism and of one cultural system coexisting. As mentioned above, this is not the result of cultural assimilation; rather mixed partners have shared the same culture from the start. Intergenerational transmission of both language systems tends to be the prevailing pattern of upbringing, so children in Slovene–Italian marriages are bilingual. Moreover, as discussed further below, they see themselves as having two ethnic identities – Slovene and Italian – rather than having one national affiliation.

Slovene–ex-Yugoslavian mixed families

Ethnically mixed families amongst members of Slovene ethnicity and immigrant groups from ex-Yugoslav republics present a rather different picture. There are active assimilation processes in favour of the Slovene language and culture, resulting in a tendency to monolingualism and, simultaneously, the prevalence of more or less distinctive cultural pluralism. This pattern stands for interpartner relations only, with intergenerational transmission of cultural elements and language revealing a primacy of Slovene language and culture. Assimilation processes in favour of the dominant language/culture for children born into mixed marriages between Slovenes and members of immigrant groups are more obvious. Family unity acts as a means of assimilating immigrant groups into dominant Slovene culture.

Consequently, in their daily communications with other people as well as within their family, children use only the Slovene language. Nonetheless, such children tend to have some level of competence in the non-Slovene language and use it with their relatives from other former Yugoslav republics. Moreover, children living in this type of mixed family largely declare themselves to be Slovenes rather than identifying with two national affiliations.

Across the two sorts of mixed partners and families, the cultural elements that seem to be most important are those that are so stable and resistant that they constantly remind the partners of their culturally mixed marriage. As such, they can be a potential source of chronic disagreement and conflict. Most problematic in this regard tend to be differences in the perception and expectations of gender roles. This is especially so for marriages between Slovenes and immigrants; and where the man (not the woman) comes from a culture with a more traditional and patriarchal orientation (e.g., a Slovene woman married to a Muslim man from Bosnia). Such embedded cultural confrontations affect the partners' satisfaction with life in a mixed family.

Satisfaction with life in a mixed family

Earlier research on cross-ethnic partnering argued that such marriages are less stable and lasting than homogamous ones (Merton 1941; Gordon 1964). The additional need for intercultural adjustment of expectations, and the negative attitude of the broader family and ethnic group are believed to influence the (dis)satisfaction of partners.

The level of satisfaction with life in an ethnically mixed marriage/family varied among the Slovene Istria respondents in my study. Yet, there was a tendency towards satisfaction. The partners point out that their decision to enter into a mixed marriage was based on love and that love is more important than cultural determinants such as religion or national affiliation or the opinion of the broader society. However, the factors that lower satisfaction with marital life, as mentioned earlier, are self-perceived intercultural differences and in particular major differences in expectations concerning gender roles, intimate life and so on, as illustrated in the following quotations:

> Sometimes he'd say, "wife, in Bosnia you wouldn't do this". I'd say, "I don't care, I'm in Slovenia, not down there". Well, if I stayed home it'd be different. As I work, my husband can't just come home and have his lunch ready. Eventually, we'll eat, if not at six, we'll eat at seven or eight. This is normal everywhere where women work. I think it's hard, really.
>
> (Slovene female, 38)

> Our ways of thinking don't get along. The system of all Bosnian mums is to teach their child that she's a woman, which means that she's a housewife in the first place. And let's say you go to work, so when you come home you want to eat! But there's nothing to eat. That's a shame, why have a wife then! But wait, you know what you got to do, you know your share of work in the house. It's normal that I expect my wife to cook for me. Me, for example, no way would I do anything. I'd go to an inn to eat. Simple.
>
> (Bosnian male, 38)

The second factor that can lower the degree of satisfaction with marital life is the presence of nationalism, particularly when it is oriented towards children or partner:

> I say to my little daughter, "if someone says something to you, say that you're a baštardo,[4] because your mother is Slovene and your father from Bosnia down there, I'm a baštardo." Now she got used to it, but it was hard at the beginning. "Mum, they told me I'm Bosnian." "Yes, fine, and you tell them they are dum yokels."
>
> (Slovene female, 34)

Finally, greater intercultural differences mean that the level of satisfaction with marital life is a less stable category in families where one of the partners is a member of an immigrant group. In Slovene–Italian families there is a high degree of satisfaction with life in a mixed family with the exception of those families in which the Slovene partner comes from other areas of Slovenia and does not speak the Italian language (predominantly the case in Slovene Istria). In these families, conflicts and dissatisfaction concentrate around linguistic issues. The response and interference of relatives or extended families can also prove problematic:

> For instance, my husband says that whenever he hears us talking [wife and children in Italian], he feels like a foreigner. He feels like a foreigner in his own family, because in fact we don't speak his language. I don't know. Maybe, that's true. But when I hear them talking in Slovene I don't feel like a foreigner.
>
> (Italian female, 43)

In situations where there is conflict and crisis, it is women who tend to assume the more active role in the process of stabilizing a family life, adapting to the needs of their partner. For instance, they may enroll on a course to learn their husband's language, they can agree to give their son an Italian name to fulfil their husband's wish even though the name is used for women in the Slovene context, and they may raise their children in their husband's religion (Sedmak 2002a, 2002b).

Extended family responses

The response of extended family to one of their members embarking on an ethnically mixed marriage implicitly reflects broader social attitudes towards a defined ethnic group and consequently towards cross-ethnic partnerships. The most frequent advice that parents gave their children upon entering a mixed marriage included accepting statements such as: "Whatever you choose you will have" and "It's your life, you know best." Nevertheless, some partners also reported that, "despite never saying or doing anything concrete, they (wider family) had their own ideas" about the national affiliation of their partner.

The cultural, geographical and social proximity between the Slovene and Italian autochthonous ethnicities and the historical presence of the Italian culture and language in Slovene Istria are evident, with the response of extended family members of the Slovene partner to an ethnically mixed marriage with a member of the Italian minority being relatively positive. Marriage to an autochthonous Italian was viewed as marriage to a local, or "one of us":

> No, I think they actually liked it. For instance, my parents went to school under Italian Zone B and they knew Italian. And my dad's parents and his whole family lived in Sečovlje until 1938, I think, so they only spoke the Trieste dialect. Yes, yes, their response was positive. I think they liked it that I got a local.
>
> (Slovene female, 45)

Nevertheless, this acceptance largely applies to local or autochthonous family-kinship networks that share the experience of the coexistence of Slovene and Italian ethnicities, as well as knowledge of the Italian and Slovene languages.

The response of extended family members who come from continental Slovenia can be less tolerant:

> But we had big fights back then, because my husband suddenly asked me why I didn't want to speak Slovene. This is how he saw it, that I didn't want to speak Slovene. I said, "No problem, my child speaks both anyway." But the problem wasn't my husband; I found that out only years later. The problem was his family, they were afraid that the poor child wouldn't learn Slovene.
>
> (Italian female, 43)

Families of the partners in mixed marriages between Slovenes and members of immigrant groups from former Yugoslavia displayed a greater variety of responses. These ranged from complete refusal through neutral acceptance to a very positive attitude towards a new family member of a different ethnic origin. Where family members were employed in public administration, the army, customs, police and so on, they often expressed a more favourable attitude towards ethnically mixed marriages of their members. Their attitude is not surprising: these services were permeated with the ideology of the common Yugoslav ethnic affiliation, ethnic equality and the common Serbo-Croatian language that was supposed to neutralize interethnic differences:

> My father was an army officer. He served in the Yugoslav army. And there were Croats and Serbs in the army. My parents displayed great national consciousness not only as Slovenes, also as Yugoslavs, and that's why it didn't bother them. To marry a German, that would've been another story. But I married a Yugoslav and that was fine.
>
> (Slovene female, 49)

There is a gendered dimension to extended family responses. Negative attitudes are often inspired by fear and concern on the part of Slovene parents in relation to their daughters entering into a mixed marriage with a foreigner (but not their sons!):

> Then my mum started bugging me, like "Don't you know his mentality, after all he's from down there." She wasn't impressed. She was simply afraid that he would convince me and take me down there and if something went wrong, he would take my children away from me and take them in Bosnia. She just didn't trust them.
>
> (Slovene female, 36)

Nonetheless, where it existed, initial intolerance among the members of the broader family usually faded, and was followed by inclusion of the new family member – belonging to a different ethnic affiliation – into the network of family-kinship relations.

Children's views

Generally, children themselves accept the cultural, linguistic, religious and other mixtures characterizing their parents as given, unquestionable and unproblematic, within their families. But their lives also encompass broader kinship networks, their neighbourhood, their peers and the general social context. My research in Slovene Istria (Sedmak 2002a, 2003a, 2006) confirms the results of studies carried out in other cultural environments, which show that the potential issues children born into ethnically mixed families have to confront – concerning self-declaration of nationality, identity construction, shame of a "wrong" surname or "wrong" affiliation of their father or mother – are the result of intolerant and nationalist attitudes in their environment, rather than intrinsic to the ethnic diversity of their parents *per se* (Cerroni-Long 1985; Romano 1988; Augustin 1989; Waldren 1998).

The generally higher level of tolerance towards and acceptance of members of the Italian minority expressed by Slovenes also applies to children born into Slovene–Italian mixed families. These children perceive their position as unproblematic; they are bilingual (without exception) and proud of it, and they regard the different origins of their parents as "normal and self-evident". A significant feature of these children's identity is that they do not see themselves monoethnically – as solely Slovene or Italian. When forced into exclusive declarations of nationality in formal situations, such as population, school and municipal censuses, they often resort to supranational declarations such as citizen of the World or member of the human race, or refuse to declare a national affiliation:

> I'm a child of the world. I have no national awareness, no feeling of affiliation, and no religion.
>
> (Daughter of Slovene–Italian parents, 18)

> I simply did not declare. There was only one answer possible followed by a possibility not to declare and that's what I chose to underline.
>
> (Daughter of Slovene–Italian parents, 19)

The perceptions of children born into mixed marriages of Slovenes and members of other nations of former Yugoslavia are more complex. Reflecting the relatively uniform response of their parents (see above), these children had a clear tendency towards monoethnic declaration – "I'm Slovene" – and towards the exclusive use of the Slovene language in public and family communication.

Children may either accept the fact of being Slovene to the extent that they can "forget" the nationality of their immigrant parent, or feel ashamed of the nationality of their immigrant parent and therefore more or less intentionally attribute little importance to it by explicitly emphasizing their Slovenehood:

> My daughter comes from school and says: "Dad, do you know that that guy is a Croat?" Then my husband says: "Do you know that your dad is a Croat, too?" And she says: "My dad is not a Croat!"
>
> (Slovene female, 49)

Parents often want to teach their children about their ethnically mixed origins and to explain the positive aspects of their family's ethnic backgrounds. Nonetheless, most leave the decision of national affiliation to their children and do not force them into exclusive declarations.

Impact of social and political circumstances

Social-political changes affecting Slovenia in the last decade of the twentieth century, notably the disintegration of former Yugoslavia, Slovenian independence and the phenomenon of new borders, have shaped the identity and everyday life of members of ethnically mixed families (Sedmak 2002b).

The already mentioned involuntary status shift from intranational ethnically mixed marriages into international ones, burdened members of mixed families with new stressful situations and the need to find survival strategies for their altered circumstances. The status shift is reflected in various fields in the everyday life of ethnically mixed families, especially for those families consisting of Slovenes and members of other nationalities of former Yugoslavia. In addition to the usual processes of intercultural coexistence, further stressful situations were faced, with the most frequent being:

- temporary or permanent interruption of contacts with wider family and problems related to the maintenance of previous contacts between members of their extended family;
- often unpleasant procedures for the acquisition of Slovene citizenship;
- increased nationalism and xenophobia in society;
- conflict relations in the macro-politics of social life pervading the micro level of family life.

In these altered socio-political circumstances, individuals living in mixed families had to cope with problems outside and within their families. Extra-familial problems manifested themselves in the increasing nationalism and xenophobic intolerance expressed by the Slovene population in their attitude towards foreigners, different cultures and languages. This increase can be placed in the context of wider processes of identification and differentiation in Slovene society. The period after independence has been followed by restoration and legitimization of the Slovene ethnic identity, with attempts to mark a clear division in relation to other ethnic groups. Consequently there are explicit emphases on cultural and language purity and more or less evident expressions of violence in relation to those deviating from such ideals, notably towards those immigrants who could not or did not want to assimilate linguistically:

> When we came to Slovenia, the situation was completely different. The language was not considered so much. We could understand each other. Now, with this war, it's totally different, right? You're being looked down on because of the way you speak. It was not like that before.
>
> (Bosnian female, 35)

The phenomenon of "Serbian collective guilt", whereby all those of Serbian nationality are held responsible for the situation and the war in the Balkans, can also be included among extra-familial forms of violence. The burden of "Serbian collective guilt" also affects family members of Serbian immigrants:

> When it started, it went on non-stop for quite some time. At work and coming from the people who in fact don't know anything, who probably have never been outside the Slovene territory. I think this was the reason why they reacted and thought this way. I tried to ignore banter and avoid it, because it was easier that way. I couldn't fight with them and make them understand that not all Serbs are enemies and bad guys, they don't all commit atrocities. My husband, too, automatically he was the bad guy, and so was my family. I couldn't make them understand that I've never had any conflicts in Serbia, that nobody has insulted me, that nobody has ever humiliated or degraded me.
>
> (Slovene female, 40)

Other, more hidden and perhaps less common problems manifesting within families stem from the dynamics of split loyalties, exclusive ethnic affiliation and intra-family nationalism, resulting in hostility from one family member towards other family members for their "wrong" or different ethnic affiliation. Parents are particularly stricken by intolerance in relation to their children:

> We've never had problems because I'm a Muslim and my husband a Slovene. But in fact, before the independence of Slovenia, it had all started already back then, my children asked me who they were. They said, "Mother, will you be mad if we say we're Slovenes like Dad?"
>
> (Bosnian female, 54)

It has to be pointed out, however, that the problem of split loyalty emerges only when people are faced with explicit demands for national identification. Many in mixed marriages believe that the phenomenon of double ethnicity did not previously provoke any problems or doubts. What follows is a quotation from a Slovene woman whose husband, a nationally conscious Serb, in her words, did not want to apply for Slovene citizenship because of his stubbornness and pride, which placed her in a sticky situation. He did not have Slovene citizenship and explicitly expressed his support for the then nationalist Serbian leader Slobodan Miloševič. As a consequence, he lost his job and could not get a new one, which led to a critical family economic situation and subsequent couple and family conflict. The situation deteriorated with the children's disagreement with their father's political conviction. The couple's son and daughter identified themselves as Slovenes:

> I tell him, "Now go to Milošević, he'll give you your pension." Yes, yes, he was foolish and he ruined us and himself for politics. All of us resent that. Look, now he's nobody! If only he had been just a bit smarter. But he ruined everything for his ideals, because he was stubborn. Yes, he was sorry later on, but then it was too late.
>
> (Slovene female, 48)

Members of ethnically mixed families respond to stressful situations by establishing various survival strategies to deal with their altered social circumstances. Confrontations with extra-family nationalism created a tendency to adopt the Slovene language for everyday communication in order to avoid the nationalistic intolerance expressed towards linguistically non-assimilated immigrants. This use of the Slovene language as an essential means of communication often was prompted by the Slovene partner:

> And I said, "Look," I said, "Mirko, learn to speak Slovene as soon as you can, or they'll have you for a Bosnian and will regard you suspiciously." Unfortunately, that's how it is, here.
>
> (Slovene female, 42)

An example of the adoption of a "language survival strategy" is provided by a father who wanted to protect his daughters from possible expressions of nationalistic intolerance: he changed the final -ć in their surname into a -č on their school certificates and other documents. The letter -ć does not exist in the Slovene alphabet and is therefore a visible sign of non-Slovene ethnicity.

For crisis situations within families, the most frequent survival strategy adopted is the avoidance of problematic conversation topics, usually related to politics and the political situation, questions of responsibility and guilt for the war and the present situation:

> In our home we simply put it away. He is watching these political things, he is following them, but I put it all aside, I don't want to deal with it. No. I never express any opinion related to that. I can have my opinion but that shouldn't affect my family. I won't allow that. I consciously pushed away politics and I'm not interested in it at all. It can endanger the existence of my family.
>
> (Slovene female, 40)

As one interviewee put it: Politics is one thing, life is another!

Concluding remarks

How members of mixed families view their situation, and their subsequent levels of satisfaction with life in a mixed family, is not given or unchangeable; rather their perceptions are shaped by a number of factors, notably:

- the environment in which a mixed family lives (multicultural, monocultural, tolerant, racist, xenophobic, etc.);
- the culture, religion, race, and/or linguistic group to which members of mixed families belong (dominant, with higher status, deprived, minority group, etc.);
- the context of political and historical circumstances in which a mixed family lives (social stability, economic prosperity, war, state border changes, etc.);
- the way that a racial, cultural, religious, linguistic ethnic group perceives cross-ethnic partnership (norms of homogeneity, permeable boundaries, etc.); and
- last but not least, the views and responses of extended family to one of their members entering into a mixed marriage.

The influence of these factors on the everyday life of members of a mixed family also varies according to the importance given to it by all involved. I conclude with the thoughts of a man with direct experience in family mixing:

> Love surpasses nationality!
>
> (Croat male, 49)

Notes

1 According to the last population census conducted in 2002, Slovenia is more than 83 per cent Slovene and 7.4 per cent other ethnic groups. The missing percentiles consist of residents who declared themselves regionally or did not want to declare ethnically (9.6 per cent).

2 The presented results are based on the two pieces of research conducted in the area of Slovene Istra in the period from 1999 to 2007. The first one included 144 adults (or 72 couples) living in ethnically mixed marriages, selected with a combination of social networking and snowball strategy. The second was conducted among 45 secondary school pupils with an exclusive experience as a "mixed" child. Children were selected randomly. In the first study the combined methodological approach involved a questionnaire and the collection of auto/biographical stories, while in the second case a structured questionnaire was used.

3 Beforehand it had been a part of the Austro-Hungarian Empire.

4 A mongrel dog, of unknown rather than mixed ancestry.

References

Augustin, B. (1989) *Marriage Across Frontiers*, Bristol: WBC Print Ltd.

Breger, R. and Hill, R. (1998) "Introducing Mixed Marriages". In R. Breger and R. Hill (eds) *Cross-Cultural Marriage*, Oxford, New York: Berg, 1–32.

Cerroni-Long, E.L. (1985) "Marrying Out: Socio-Cultural and Psychological Implications of Intermarriage". In G. Kurian (ed.) *Journal of Comparative Family Studies. Special Issue: Intermarriage*, 16, 1: 25–46.

Darovec, D. (2008) *Kratka zgodovina Istre* [*A Short Hystory of Istria*], Koper: Založba Annales.

Elias, N. and Scotson, J.L. (1994) *The Established and the Outsider*, London, Thousand Oaks, CA, New Delhi: SAGE Publications.

Eriksen, Th.H. (1993) *Ethnicity and Nationalism: Anthropological Perspectives*, London, Chicago: Pluto Press.

Gordon, A.I. (1964) *Intermarriage: Interfaith, Interracial, Interethnic*, Boston: Beacon Press.

Ibrahim, F.A. and Schroeder, D.G. (1990) "Cross-Cultural Couples Counseling: A Developmental, Psychoeducational Intervention". In G. Kurian (ed.) *Journal of Comparative Family Studies. Special Issue: Intermarriage*, 21, 2: 193–205.

Merton, R.K. (1941) "Intermarriage and the Social Structure: Fact and Theory", *Psychiatry*, 4: 361–74.

Mikolič, V. (2003a) "Makro in mikro struktura družbenega odnosa do italijanske manjšinske skupnosti in dvojezičnosti v slovenski Istri" ["Macro and Micro Structure of Social Attitudes Towards the Italian Minority and Bilingualism in Slovene Istria"], *Annales, Series Historia et Sociologia*, 13, 2: 373–88.

—(2003b) *Jezik kot odraz etnične ozaveščenosti v narodnostno mešanem prostoru slovenske Istre* [*Language as a Reflection of Ethnic Awareness in the Nationally Mixed Territory of Slovene Istria*], Ljubljana: Katedra za slovenski jezik in stilistiko, Filozofska fakulteta.

Romano, D. (1988) *Intercultural Marriage, Promises & Pitfalls*, Boston: Intercultural Press Inc.

Sedmak, M. (2002a) *Kri in kultura: Etnično mešane zakonske zveze v slovenski Istri* [*Blood and Culture: Ethnically Mixed Marriages in Slovene Istria*], Koper: Založba Annales.

—(2002b) "The Changeable Status: Transformation of Intranational Ethnically Mixed Marriages into International Ones", *Društvena Istraživanja*, 62: 971–94.

——(2003a) "Dinamika kulturnih in identitetnih medgeneracijskih transmisij pri otrocih etnično mešanih družin" ["Dynamics of Cultural and Identity Intergenerational Transmissions in Children of Ethnically Mixed Families"], *Annales, Series Historia et Sociologia*, 13, 1: 71–86.

——(2003b) "Stališča mladih slovenske Istre do (med)kulturnih fenomenov okolja bivanja" ["Stances of the Youth of Slovene Istria Towards (Inter)Cultural Phenomena in Their Living Environment"], *Annales, Series Historia et Sociologia*, 13, 2: 405–24.

——(2006) "Etnično mešane družine" ["Ethnically Mixed Families"]. In T. Rener *et al.* (eds) *Družine in družinsko življenje v Sloveniji*. Koper: Založba Annales, 191–221.

——(2009) "Izzivi medkulturnosti" ["A Challenge of Interculturalism"]. In M. Sedmak (ed.) *Podobe obmejnosti*. Koper: Založba Annales, 13–36.

Sedmak, M., Furlan, M. and Mikolič, V. (2002a) *Ekonomski položaj italijanske manjšine v Sloveniji* [*Economic Position of the Italian Minority in Slovenia*], Koper: ZRS Koper, Center za pospeševanje podjetništva Piran.

——(2002b) *Identiteta slovenske Istre* [*Identity of Slovene Istria*], Koper: ZRS Koper.

Štrukelj, I. (1986) *Mešani zakoni: sociološke in socialno-psihološke razsežnosti narodne eksogamije in jezikovne heterogamije* [*Mixed Marriages: Social and Psychological Implications*], Ljubljana: Inštitut za sociologijo.

Sussi, E. (1994) *I matrimoni misti nel Friuli-Venezia Gulia* [*Ethnically Mixed Marriages in Friuli-Venezia Gulia*], Pula: Pedagoski fakultet.

Waldren, J. (1998) "Crossing Over: Mixing, Matching and Marriage in Mallorca". In R. Breger and R. Hill (eds) *Cross-Cultural Marriage*, Oxford, New York: Berg, 33–48.

6 Constructing multiraciality in US families and neighbourhoods

Steven R. Holloway, Richard Wright and Mark Ellis

Introduction

The racial categorization systems used by the United States Census until the mid-1990s forced people to report race (or have their race reported for them) in singular and mutually exclusive categories. Under pressure from various groups, the US Office of Management and Budget (1997) instituted the new "mark one or more" system of racial classification designed to accommodate the racial claims of multiracial people in time for the 2000 Census (Perlmann and Waters 2002; Williams 2006). This taxonomic shift lays bare the social construction of race at the national scale. This chapter examines the construction of race, in particular multiraciality, at more local levels: by families in neighbourhoods. Specifically, we ask what happens when parents of multiracial children are allowed to mark more than one category on the Census form. What are the sorts of neighbourhood where mixed-race couples are most apt to identify their children as multiracial on the Census? Does neighbourhood racial diversity affect the likelihood of this choice? Will the whiteness of neighbourhoods be reflected in the whiteness of choices mixed-race couples make when identifying their children? Will the "some other race" option retain its salience in certain contexts? This chapter provides empirical answers to these questions based on an analysis of confidential 2000 Census data.

Our study connects two recent streams of research. First, several researchers utilized individual-level US Census 2000 data to explore the emergence of multiraciality (e.g., Bratter 2007; Liebler 2010; Roth 2005) examining the likelihood that parents of multiracial children classified (or reported) their children with multiple racial categories. Each analysis had a particular goal and each accounted for local context in some way. They conceptualized the impacts differently but all found that local context mattered, typically with multiracial children more likely to be reported with multiple racial categories when families live in places where multiracial populations concentrate. All these investigations, however, were forced to measure contextual racial composition using large geographic units with at least 100,000 people. Local neighbourhood effects in the 2000 Census, for example at the census-tract scale, remain unexplored.

Holloway *et al.* (2009) provide the only neighbourhood-scale analysis of the racial claims made for children in mixed-race families. With only single-race choices available for analysis in 1990, their study leveraged mixed-race parentage to study local variation in the racial claims these couples made for their multiracial children. They found that mixed-race couples were more likely to report their children as white when they lived in white neighbourhoods and more apt to report a non-white category when they lived in non-white neighbourhoods. Intriguingly, parents of some multiracial children became more likely to report a category other than one of their own two categories when they lived in racially diverse neighbourhoods, primarily through the Census-provided option of "some other race", though this effect was statistically significant only for children in white–black mixed-race households.

Now that the US Census allows the marking of multiple racial categories, we re-open the question of how the act of claiming race for multiracial children relates to the racial configuration of neighbourhood contexts. We understand this relationship as mutual and reciprocal – that is, families more likely to conceive of their children as multiracial may also be more likely to live in certain kinds of racially configured neighbourhoods, while at the same time certain kinds of neighbourhoods likely influence the way that parents conceive of and/or report their children's racial identity. While our empirical information does not allow us to sort out in which direction the causal arrow points most strongly, we frame our discussion and analysis by focusing on the ways that multiraciality emerges at multiple scales. We ground this investigation in a conceptual framework that stresses the importance of racial diversity, conceived of at three main scales: the body, the family, and the neighbourhood. Before discussing our framework, however, we review existing research.

Geographic context and multiraciality

Geographies play into assessments of multiraciality and the choices people make or have made for them (e.g., Mahtani 2002; Holloway *et al.* 2009; Clark and Maas 2009; Johnston *et al.* 2006; Bratter and Heard 2009). For example, David Brunsma (2005) concluded that the interactions among gender, class, and context mediate the racial identification of multiracial children. In a related study, Wendy Roth (2005) focused on the racial categories reported for children from black/non-black interracial marriages using the 5 per cent Public Use Microdata Sample (PUMS) from the 2000 US Census. She was particularly interested in multiracial individuals with black heritage and the lasting effects of the so-called "one drop rule" that socially and legally codified anyone with any kind of African background as "black" (Hollinger 2005; Khanna 2010). Controlling for Census Division (region), her models included two racial composition variables measured on the basis of large geographic areas (Public Use Microdata Areas, or PUMAs, which house at least 100,000 people): the percentage black and the share of the area's total population that is black-and-white. She found that in these black/non-black households, multiracial children were more likely to be classified by their parents as black only, and less likely to be classified as white only or white-and-black, when they lived in geographic areas characterized by a large black population. Conversely, when they lived in places where the multiracial share of total population is large, parents were more likely to categorize their child using a racial category other than black. Specifically, the odds of identifying a child as white–black grew in areas with elevated numbers of people who claimed to be black-and-white.

Jennifer Bratter's (2007) primary focus was on the impact of mixed-race parents on the racial classification of multiracial children. She organized the Census data into four groups defined by type of mixed-race family: white/non-white, black/non-black, Asian/non-Asian, and American Indian/non-American Indian. For each of these groups except American Indians, living in a place with larger shares of population reported with multiple racial categories significantly predicts a greater likelihood that parents opt for multicategory racial classification for their multiracial children.

Carolyn Liebler (2010) explored patterns of multiraciality among American Indians who were intermarried and lived with their spouse and child(ren). She distinguished between what she called social context (i.e., the spaces of home and the family) and physical context, which she specifically defined as indigenous homelands that carry cultural meaning. Controlling for family ties and socio-economic status as well as the area's racial composition, she found a clear relationship between residence on an American Indian homeland and the child's chances of being reported as single-race American Indian. She joins others, such as Khanna (2010), who observe that despite the dawning of a multiracial new day, the intergenerational transmission of strong and singular identities continues in the context of places freighted with cultural meaning.

Framing multiraciality

Our conceptual framework builds on Holloway *et al.* (2009), which theorized processes of racial formation as multiply scaled and geographically contextual. We specifically argued that racial formation operates not just at the scale of the nation-state (Omi and Winant 1994; Goldberg 2002), but also at the scales of neighbourhood and household. The act of parents marking racial categories on behalf of multiracial children – that is, making racial claims – for us represented a complex and contingent racial socialization that both reflected and shaped neighbourhood racial configurations. Drawing on theory that posited the active constitutive role of space and place in racialized social processes (e.g., Delaney 2002), we argued that there may be a matching of neighbourhood-level compositional diversity with the choice to mark children as neither white nor non-white.

> The composite racial identity of a place (i.e. not white, but also not singly black or Latino or Asian, etc.) associates with the composite racial identity of a multiracial child as not white and simultaneously not black, Latino or Asian. We are agnostic about the causal ordering of the association – it is certainly possible that families who imagine their children's racial identity as composite will be drawn to live in places with a composite racial identity just as it is also possible that living in a diverse place may encourage parents to think of their children as outside the binary either/or categorization typically employed.
>
> (Holloway *et al.* 2009, p. 529)

Two changes guide us to extend and deepen our thinking in this chapter. First, the empirical results of our analysis of 1990 data were supportive of our understanding of the relationship between racial claims and neighbourhood context, but not overwhelmingly so. Children in white–black households were more often reported as "some other race" in our study when their families lived in racially diverse neighbourhoods. While this result was consistent with our expectations, the impact of neighbourhood racial diversity on racial claims outside the binary categorization was more ambiguous for children in white–Asian and white–Latino/a households. Second, changes in the racial reporting rules in the 2000 US Census make forms of racial diversity not observable in our analysis of 1990 Census data statistically legible for the first time.

In our previous study (Holloway *et al.* 2009), we understood the option of marking "some other race" as likely indicative of a rejection of the binary single-category options available on the 1990 Census form. The new mark-one-or-more option of racial classification allows parents to directly escape the confines of either/or classification. The racial claims made by parents on behalf of their multiracial children are meaningful acts of racial identification (Rockquemore, Brunsma and Delgado 2009) that reflect, if only imperfectly, their understanding of who their children are racially, as well as who they may want their children to become racially. The choice to mark multiple racial categories thus must be understood as a claim of bodily racial diversity distinct from the alternative choices of marking a single racial category. This explicitly multiracial form of racial diversity attaches to the scale of the body, as reported by parents on the Census form. We do not contend that the act of a parent reporting her child's racial categories on a Census is indicative or formative of the child's "true" racial identity. Moreover, children will be racially identified by many people in multiple ways and will likely develop situationally flexible personal racial identities over their life course, and our analysis cannot be predictive of these developments. Even so, the act of claiming race on behalf of a multiracial child does inform us about how and where multiraciality can be conceived of within families.

The multiraciality that became legible with the change in official US data collection practices also forces us to reconceive the racial configuration of neighbourhoods. In Holloway *et al.* (2009), we focused on an aggregate and general form of compositional diversity, asserting that racially diverse neighbourhoods comprised a racial configuration distinct from the singly raced types of segregated racialized neighbourhoods more typically imagined in US metropolitan contexts – that is, diverse neighbourhoods are neither predominantly white nor predominantly black. Subsequent to that analysis we have come to recognize that there are multiple forms of neighbourhood-level diversity (Holloway *et al.* 2012; www.mixedmetro.com) that both enfold and are enfolded by the more stereotypical understandings of segregated neighbourhoods. Holloway *et al.* (2012) begin to differentiate compositionally diverse neighbourhoods according to which racial group remains in the plurality. Here, we take our cue from the recent studies that find an association between large geographic areas with a relatively large share of multiracial population and parents' racial classification of their multiracial children (Bratter 2007; Liebler 2010; Roth 2005). In sum, places in which multiracial people (i.e., people who mark or have marked for them multiple racial categories on the Census form) concentrate potentially signify a new kind of racialized diversity with distinct geographic expression that we are just beginning to comprehend.

Frey and Myers (2002) computed residential segregation indices for US cities and metropolitan areas using 2000 Census data. They found that the population reporting two or more races is less residentially segregated, on average, than the single race population. Clark and Maas (2009) document some of the distinct geographic patterns associated with specific multiracial types for metropolitan areas in California. Both studies optimistically argue that multiracial people are more spatially integrated, and thus assimilated, with whites than single race non-white populations. The maps displayed in Clark and Maas (2009), however, portray a spatial pattern whereby multiracial people in California metropolitan areas concentrate in neighbourhoods geographically distinct from both white and non-white populations. We build on these suggestive findings to portray our conceptualization and measurement of the neighbourhood concentration of multiracial people as a potentially distinct spatial form of racialized diversity.

In summary, our conceptual framework contends that multiraciality should be understood as an emergent and newly legible form of racialized diversity that operates simultaneously at the scales of the body, the family, and the neighbourhood. Moreover, multiraciality at one scale of expression affects its expression at the other scales. We thus expect that the neighbourhood concentration of multiracial people will contextually influence the choices that mixed-race couples make about how to report the race of their multiracial children. Specifically, we expect that residence in such racially diverse neighbourhoods will be associated with an elevated likelihood that parents will mark multiple racial categories. Our framework resonates with the mixed-race theoretical tradition that Rockquemore, Brunsma and Delgado (2009) describe as *ecological* because it asserts that neighbourhood contexts can affect expressions of multiraciality. Even so, our conceptual and empirical focus remains on the multiply scaled expression of this emergent form of racial diversity.

Data and analysis

Our analysis uses confidential individual- and family-level data from the 2000 US Census. We selected 16 large metropolitan areas for study to balance the goals of regional representation, a variety of economic bases, and being able to work with large enough samples (these Census data are based on a 1-in-6 sample of housing units).To facilitate our examination of racial claims made on behalf of children in mixed-race households, we selected households with an adult male and an adult female reported as either cohabiting or married. These households must also have a child less than five years old. This restriction increases the chances that the child is the biological offspring of the adults. It also reduces the time-frame in which the household could have moved since the birth of the child. This reduces though does not eliminate the risk of endogeneity between a child's phenotypic appearance and the household's residential location. For example, by restricting our sample to pre-school aged children, we reduce the probability that a household with a multiracial child with dark skin tone and/or tightly curly hair has relocated to a segregated non-white neighbourhood specifically in the hope of avoiding having their child be treated as racially distinct from peers in segregated white neighbourhoods.

We further restrict our analysis to households that define themselves on Census forms as headed by white–black and white–Asian couples. The United States broadly defines as "Asian" any individual with East, Southeast, and South Asian ancestry. It is not possible with our data to distinguish between these sub-groups, as it is with UK data. We do include reported country of origin variables in some of our analysis. While there are many more white–Latino mixed-race households, our empirical analysis is greatly complicated by practice of the Census to collect data on Latino "ethnicity" with a question separate from that related to "race". We have operationally resolved this issue for adults by restricting our definition of race categories to "non-Hispanic" white, black, and Asian. As our focus here is on the racial classification of children, however, the interaction of Hispanic ethnicity with the race question creates too many possible responses and renders the empirical questions and methods distinct from those that we present here. Our choice to exclude white–Latino/a families is regrettable but mirrors choices made by, for example, Bratter (2007) and Roth (2005).

Structuring the analysis in this way produced a sample of 12,500 children, 8,071 in white–Asian households, and 4,469 in white–black households. Table 6.1 reports the racial claims made on behalf of these children aggregated across the 16 metropolitan areas. Several patterns are evident. First, the majority of children are reported multiracially in the two racial categories

Table 6.1 Racial claims made on behalf of young children in mixed-race households

Racial Claims	#	%
Children in white–Asian households		
white only	1,717	21.27
Asian only	1,078	13.36
white and Asian	4,724	58.53
all other possibilities	552	6.84
Children in white–black households		
white only	471	10.54
black only	965	21.59
white and black	2,573	57.57
all other possibilities	460	10.29

that match those reported for the adults in their household. Second, substantial numbers of the children are reported either with a single racial category matching only one of the adults in their household *or* with one or more racial categories that do not match either adult.

The share of children marked multiracially with two racial categories matching their adults is roughly the same for white–black households and white–Asian households. Just under 59 per cent of children in white–Asian households are marked as white *and* Asian, and just under 58 per cent of children in white–black households are marked as white *and* black. The share of children marked with other options, however, differs considerably between the two groups. Children in white–Asian households are much more likely overall to be marked as white only (about 21 per cent) than Asian only (about 13 per cent), with all other possibilities only rarely marked (about 7 per cent). Children in white–black households show the opposite pattern, being marked as black only almost twice as often as white only (about 22 per cent vs. 11 per cent, respectively). On the surface, this pattern is consistent with the US's long standing and apparently still socially significant "one-drop rule" of hypodescent. Notably, however, the share of children in white–black households that are not marked with any combination of white or black (about 10 per cent) is larger than for children in white–Asian households. This perhaps reflects a transgressive rejection of the use of racial categories, including the now available option of marking two categories, thus signalling multiraciality. Roth (2005) presents similar findings in her provocatively titled paper "The End of the One-Drop Rule?". She interprets this pattern as indicative of the attempt by white–black couples to reject the one-drop rule and to form a more meaningful and specifically *interracial* identity for their offspring. She argues that marking *any* category or categories other than black alone is a rejection by white–black couples of the singularity of black racial identification for their multiracial children.

To assess the possible relation between the marking of racial categories and geographic contexts, we estimated child-level multinomial logit models that include measures of a location's racial composition, including measures of multiple facets of racial diversity. We refined the spatial frame of our analysis to assess the statistical effects of local neighbourhoods on the racial identification of children. Following a long precedent in racial residential segregation and urban studies literatures, we allow census tracts to represent neighbourhoods despite the conceptual problems that accompany this choice (Martin 2003). We are able to focus in on census-tract levels of racial configuration because we had access to confidential Census data in secure research facilities. Other scholars interested in the racial contexts surrounding these processes using publicly available data (Bratter 2007; Liebler 2010; Roth 2005), by contrast, must measure "local" racial/ethnic concentrations using much larger areas of at least 100,000 residents (PUMAs) – the smallest spatial units for analysis available in that format.

To simplify the analysis and to provide analytical focus, we specified the dependent variable in these multinomial logit models as a three-category classification based on how the child was marked racially – white only, minority only (either black only or Asian only), and multiracial matching the racial categories marked for the two adults in the household (either white *and* black or white *and* Asian). This strategy includes the overwhelming majority of options recorded for the multiracial children in our sample; it excludes only those observations where the child was identified outside these three possibilities – a situation that is more difficult to account for theoretically and would complicate interpretation of the results if it were included in the model.

We identified a list of individual and child-, family-, and household-level attributes that potentially influence the racial claims made on behalf of multiracial children (Table 6.2). We added a set of metropolitan dummy variables to account for potential regional differences and a set of national ancestry dummy variables for the Asian adult in white–Asian households. We also included a set of tract-level controls: percentage of the population in active military service, median household income, percentage of adults with college education, percentage of the population older than 65, and percentage of the population currently in school. Finally, in accordance with the primary interest of this chapter, we included the following measures of neighbourhood (census-tract) racial composition: percentage white; scaled entropy as a measure of composite general neighbourhood racial diversity that takes its largest values for neighbourhoods where each of the racial groups are represented in equal shares (see Holloway *et al.* 2009 for a complete explanation of this measure); percentage foreign born; and percentage of the total population that reported two-plus races (i.e., percentage multiracial).

Neighbourhood percentage white and scaled entropy were identified in previous research as important contextual assessments in analysis of 1990 US Census data (Holloway *et al.* 2009). To these we added two measures that capture alternative facets of diversity within neighbourhoods. To acknowledge the increase in the foreign-born share of the US population in the last 50 years, and the increased share of neighbourhoods with substantial numbers of

Table 6.2 Variables included in the multinomial logit models

Child's Characteristics	**Educational Attainment**
Child's Age	Neither Partner Graduated High School
Child's Gender	Both Partners Graduated High School
Child is Foreign Born	Both with Some College
Household Characteristics	Both Graduated College
Child has Siblings in the Household	Both with Graduate or Professional Degree
English Only in the Household	Minority Partner has more Education
Minority Partner's English is Not Fluent	Minority Partner has less Education
# Persons in Housing Unit	**Work, School & Military Attachment**
Household Income	One Partner is In School
Household Income Squared	Both Partners are in School
Housing Unit is Owner Occupied	Both Partners are Retired
Household Moved from w/in Metro	Female Partner is Not In Labour Force
Household Moved from outside Metro	One or Both Partners In Military
General Characteristics of Adults	One or Both Partners Retired Military
Male Adult's Age	**Tract Racial Composition**
Parents are Married	% White
Race & Ancestry of Adults	Scaled Entropy (General Diversity)
White Adult is Male	% Multiracial
White Partner is Mixed Ancestry	% Foreign Born
Minority Partner is Mixed Ancestry	**Tract Socio-Economic Status Characteristics**
Foreign Birth Status of Adults	% Active Military
Both Partners Born in US	Median Household Income
White Partner is Foreign Born	% College Graduate
Minority Partner is Foreign Born	% > 65 Years Old
Both Partners are Foreign Born	% In School
Year of Entry Prior to 1970	Tract is in Urbanized Area
Year of Entry in 1970s	**Metropolitan Dummy Variables**
Year of Entry in 1980s	**Asian National Ancestry (Asians Only)**
Year of Entry in 1990s	

immigrants, we examined the impact of living in an immigrant residential concentration. We included neighbourhood percentage foreign born because newcomers to the US often arrive with different racial sensibilities to the native born. We suspected that residence in an immigrant neighbourhood would decrease the chances of parents reporting multiple races for their children.

Given that our central intent in this chapter is to examine the impact of multiracial neighbourhood diversity on the probability of children being marked multiracially, we included the overall share of tract population marked with two-plus racial categories (cf. Roth 2005; Liebler 2010; Bratter 2007). In preliminary analysis, we examined the possibility that young children may constitute a large share of the total population marked with multiple racial categories. We found that in the vast majority of tracts young children constitute a small share of the total multiracial population, and that the maximum share is very modest. The model estimates the effects of these four neighbourhood racial context measures on child racial identification controlling for metropolitan location and neighbourhood socioeconomic structure.

The multinomial logit models were estimated separately for children in white–black and white–Asian households, which allowed us to include the Asian ancestry variables. We built the models sequentially, adding the tract-level variables after controlling for the metropolitan area dummy variables. For both groups of multiracial children, the tract-level variables provided a statistically significant improvement to the fit of the models. In addition, the four tract variables capturing neighbourhood racial configurations were jointly significant in both models.

There are dozens of coefficients estimated by these models, which can be challenging to interpret (we will gladly make the full results available upon request). We focus our attention in this chapter on visual representations of the impacts of the four tract variables that capture neighbourhood racial configurations. Figure 6.1 shows the impact of these variables for children in white–black households and Figure 6.3 shows their impact for children in Asian–white households. Given the dependent variable's three categories, there are three types of pair-wise comparisons generated in the form of odds (e.g., the first block of bars in Figure 6.1 depicts the odds of a parent reporting black only vs. white only). The length of the bars indicates the magnitude of the effect of the tract variable on the odds – specifically, the percentage change in odds that results from a standard deviation increase in the value of the tract variable. This approach allows us to compare the magnitude of the effects across variables with different units of measurement. The figure depicts the effects directionally – bars extending to the right indicate a positive effect while bars extended to the left indicate a negative effect. Black bars indicate statistically significant effects ($p < .05$).

The racial category reported for multiracial children in white–black households is responsive to tract percentage white and percentage multiracial, regardless of the pair-wise comparison of racial categories. Based on previous research results, we had expected neighbourhood racial diversity to come into play. Here, however, the measure of general racial diversity (scaled entropy), which is maximized in neighbourhoods with equal shares of the six racial groups, does not prove to be statistically significant. In general, marking children in white–black households as black only is less likely in segregated white neighbourhoods, and marking children as multiracial is more likely in neighbourhoods where the multiracial population appears to concentrate.

Figure 6.2 presents the results in a different and perhaps more easily interpretable form. In each panel, we display predicted probability plots for the three outcome categories as influenced by the statistically significant tract-level racial composition variables (percentage white in Figure 6.2a and percentage multiracial in Figure 6.2b). The least shaded portions of these plots reflect the most commonly observed range of values for the tract variables – shaded portions of the plots reflect tract values that are rarely observed across the sample of

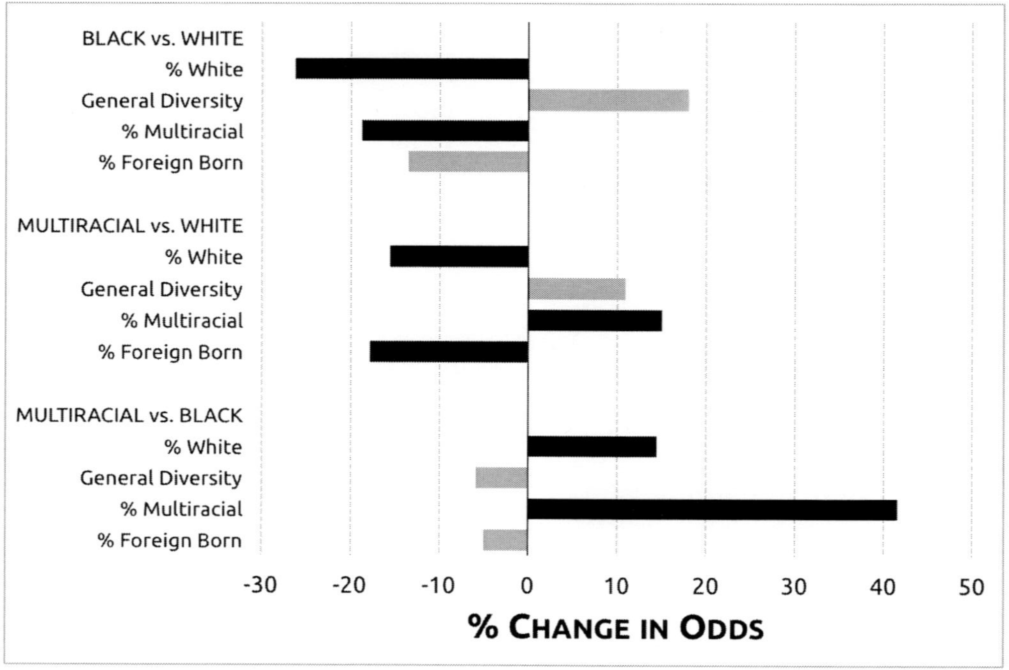

Figure 6.1 Effects of tract-level racial configuration on odds of racial reporting for children in white–black households

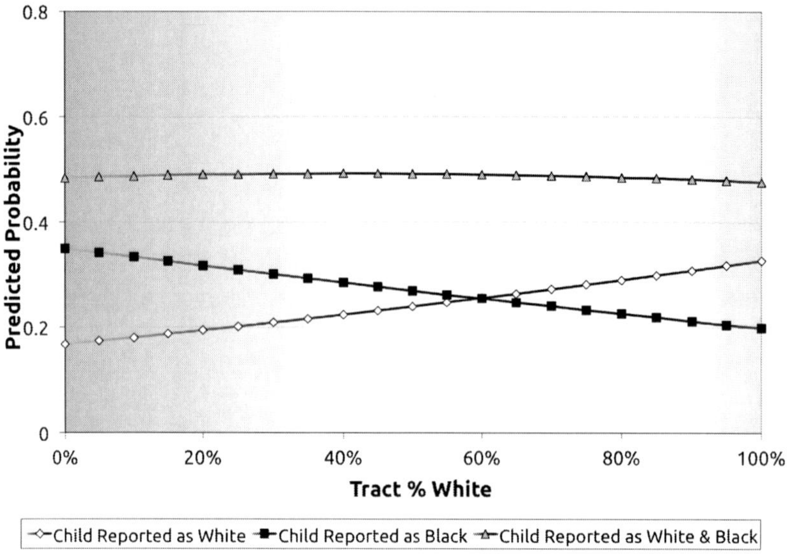

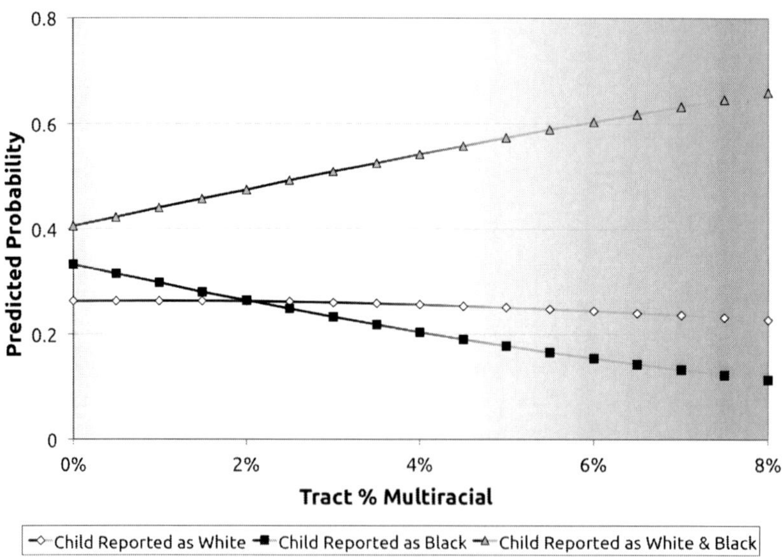

Figure 6.2 Predicted probability of racial classification in response to (6.2a) census tract percentage white and (6.2b) census tract percentage multiracial for children in white–black households

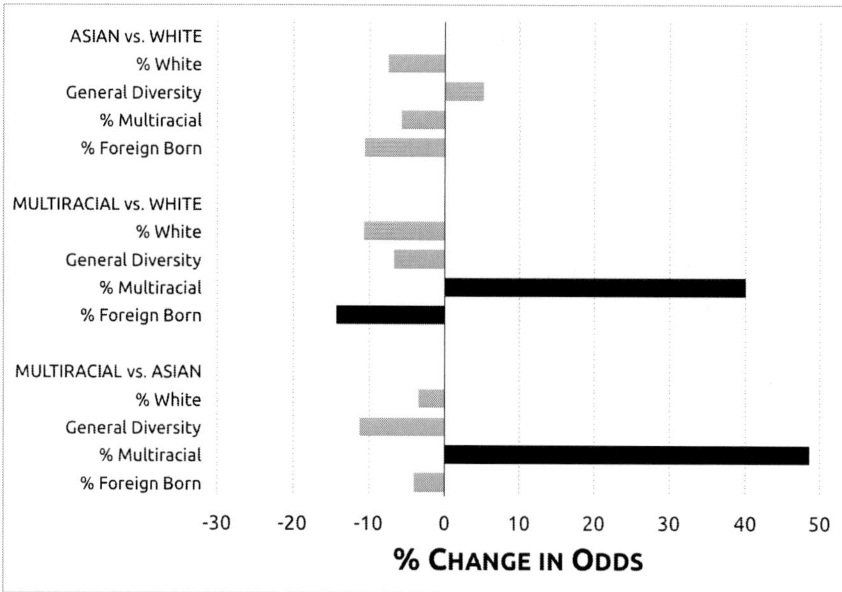

Figure 6.3 Effects of tract-level racial configuration on odds of racial reporting for children in white–Asian households

16 metropolitan areas. For children in white–black households, we see that white segregation produces a trade-off between marking white only and black only – the probability of marking both white *and* black is not affected. Neighbourhood concentrations of multiracial people, however, produce a very different pattern. Children become much more likely to be reported multiracially as black *and* white, and much less likely to be reported as white only, in neighbourhoods where multiracial people concentrate, despite the fact that the neighbourhood shares are rather small.

Figure 6.3 shows the magnitude and significance of the effects of neighbourhood racial variables on the racial classification of multiracial children in Asian–white households. Percentage multiracial has a large and positive impact on the odds of marking children as both Asian *and* white. Percentage foreign born reduces the odds of reporting children as multiracial in contrast to white only. Figure 6.4 shows these trade-offs from a different angle. In Figure 6.4a, parents become more likely to report their children as white *and* Asian as the neighbourhood percentage of the population that reports two-plus races increases, accompanied by reductions in the probability that children are reported as either white only or Asian only. The relation between racial claims and the immigrant status of neighbourhoods (Figure 6.4b) suggests that white–Asian parents become more likely to report their children as white only as the foreign-born population constitutes a larger share of the population, accompanied by reductions in the probability of claiming either Asian only or white *and* Asian.

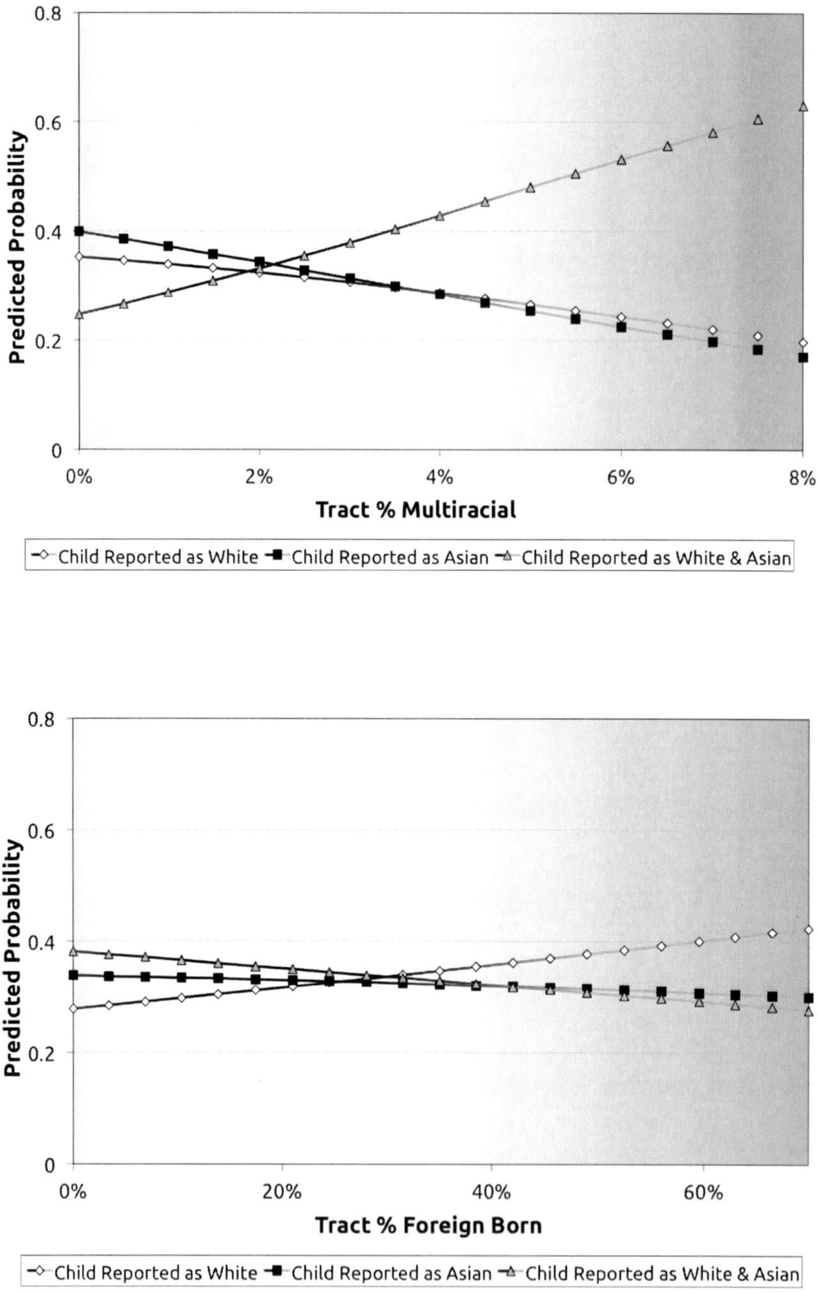

Figure 6.4 Predicted probability of racial classification in response to (6.4a) census tract percentage multiracial and (6.4b) census tract percentage foreign born for children in white–Asian households

Conclusions

Multiracial children are increasingly on the public radar in the United States. A *New York Times* article (Saulny 2011) examining the early returns from the 2010 Census (US Census Bureau 2011), for example, found that multiracial children were the fastest growing group of young people between 2000 and 2010, increasing by almost 50 per cent to more than four million. The total number of multiracial people increased by 32 per cent since 2000, with growth rates much higher in some states in the South and Midwest. The number of people marking white and black increased by a remarkable 134 per cent between 2000 and 2010. These trends highlight the importance of understanding both the forces that are promoting the formation of mixed-race romantic partners *and* the forces that affect the multiracial racial claims made on behalf of the children of these relationships. We argue that this behaviour is affected by a newly visible form of neighbourhood racial diversity; and our research findings support this argument.

Our analysis of the racial claims mixed-race couples make for their young multiracial children in 2000 indicates that many do, indeed, use the mark-more-than-one choice when filling out the US Census form. They took advantage of the new options to claim more than one race in the 2000 Census by marking the two racial categories for their children that match their own categories. We also discover, however, that a non-trivial share of parents mark only a single racial category matching one of their own racial categories, or mark one or more racial categories that do not match their own. Central to our thesis that neighbourhood context matters, our study reveals a systematic relationship between these choices and the kind of neighbourhoods in which these families live.

When young children in white–black households live in mostly segregated white neighbourhoods, their parents are apt to report them as white-only. The probability of marking a child as black *and* white is not affected by this neighbourhood characteristic. This choice is also unaffected by general neighbourhood racial diversity. In contrast, a specific and newly visible type of racial diversity – the multiracial percentage of tract population – does have a significant effect. Specifically, the probability that parents mark the multiracial option of black *and* white increases markedly as the neighbourhood share of multiracial individuals increases.

For children in white–Asian households, claiming multiraciality for children is also responsive to variations in the neighbourhood percentage of multiracial individuals; the probability that parents mark white *and* Asian increases as this form of diversity increases. Parents of white–Asian children also respond to an additional facet of diversity – the foreign-born population. As the proportion of immigrants in a neighbourhood increases, parents become more likely to mark their young multiracial children as white only, and less likely to mark them as Asian-only or white-and-Asian. The decrease in the odds of claiming a multiracial identity for their children reflects, perhaps, different sets of racial sensibilities in communities with a significant foreign-born presence. The increase in the chances of those children being identified as white captures perhaps an "assimilation-to-white" gesture by white–Asian parents in such locales.

Our focus has been on the way that neighbourhood space conditions the manner in which parents in mixed-race partnerships racially identify their young multiracial children. Multiracial neighbourhood diversity matters in these choices, suggesting a connection between the configuration of multiraciality across space at the scale of neighbourhoods and its acknowledgement within the space of the household. Multiraciality is an emergent form of diversity that is increasingly visible at the scales of the body, the family, *and* the neighbourhood. How the relationships between these spatial scales play out when children grow up and begin to assert their own identities, especially as they move away from home, is another question. Harris and Sim (2002) suggest that multiracial youth engage in situationally transient racial identification between home and school environments, depending on the immediate presence/absence of parents and peer groups. Shih, Bonam, Sanchez, and Peck (2007) find that multiracial people are much more aware that race is a social construction than are monoracial people, which may account for the contextual contingency and situational flexibility of racial self-identification. As Rockquemore, Brunsma, and Delgado (2009) stress, we recognize that the parental reporting of racial categories for small children is not the same phenomenon as racial *identity* that is developed over the children's life course. We argue, however, that since parents are reporting racial categories, our work really deals with an instance of racial *identification*. A question for future research should ask how flexible self-identifications in adolescence and early adulthood might be conditioned by diversity and racial composition in neighbourhoods and other geographic contexts experienced during early childhood. We wonder if growing up in neighbourhoods marked by multiracial diversity will promote multiracial self-identification and/or multiracial identity over the life course.

Only time will tell whether multiracial ecological settings will elevate the odds of multiracial self-identification in adulthood. If Barack Obama's decision to claim a black rather than multiracial identity on the US Census – despite being raised by a white single mother and her parents and despite growing up in Hawaii, the most diverse state in the country – is anything to go by then we should not be too eager to project that the flourishing claims of multiraciality exhibited in youth will translate into multiracial identification in adulthood. Racial hierarchy and the resultant racial stratification of key realms of life in the US unfortunately remain an enduring fact. Whiteness remains a key advantage (Lipsitz 1998) and is unlikely to fade as such in the foreseeable future in our view. To be sure, the substantial growth in the population of multiracial youth disturbs the foundation of the racial hierarchy, which may be shifting in a variety of ways to accommodate them (see Ellis 2001; Gans 1999; Bonilla-Silva 2004). The external pressures for them to fit within the single-race categories that continue to demarcate the overwhelming majority of the population will, however, be immense.

Acknowledgements

This research was made possible by grants from the National Science Foundation and the Russell Sage Foundation. Thanks to Rebecca Acosta, Angela Andrus, and Kevin McKinney at the California Census Research Data Center for assistance with the data. Thanks too to Margaret East who spent far too many hours in a small, windowless room helping with the programming and analysis. The results reported in this chapter were obtained while the authors were Census Bureau Special Sworn Status researchers. Any opinions and conclusions expressed herein are those of the authors and do not necessarily represent the views of the US Census Bureau. All results have been reviewed to ensure that no confidential information is disclosed. Support for this research at the UCLA and Berkeley Research Data Centers from the NSF (ITR-0427889) is gratefully acknowledged.

References

Anderson, M.J. (1988) *The American Census: A Social History*, New Haven: Yale University Press.

Bonilla-Silva, E. (2004) "From bi-racial to tri-racial: Towards a new system of racial stratification in the USA", *Ethnic and Racial Studies*, 27: 931–50.

Bratter, J. (2007) "Will 'multiracial' survive to the next generation? The racial classification of children of multiracial parents", *Social Forces*, 86(2): 822–49.

Bratter, J. and Heard, H. (2009) "Mother's, father's, or both? Parental gender and parent–child interactions in the racial classification of adolescents", *Sociological Forum*, 24(3): 658–88.

Brunsma, D.L. (2005) "Interracial families and the racial identification of mixed-race children: Evidence from the early childhood longitudinal study", *Social Forces*, 84(2): 1131–57.

Clark, W.A.V. and Maas, R. (2009) "The geography of a mixed-race society", *Growth and Change*, 40(4): 565–93.

Delaney, D. (2002) "The space that race makes", *Professional Geographer*, 54(1): 6–14.

Ellis, M. (2000) "'Mark one or more': Counting and projecting by race on US Census 2000 and beyond", *Social & Cultural Geography*, 1(2): 183–95.

——(2001) "What future for Whites? Population projections and racialised imaginaries in the US", *International Journal of Population Geography*, 7(3): 213–29.

Frey, W.H., and Myers, D. (2002) "Neighborhood segregation in single race and multi-race America: A census study of cities and metropolitan areas", Working Paper, Fannie Mae Foundation.

Gans, H. (1999) "The possibility of a new racial hierarchy in the twenty-first century United States". In *The Cultural Territories of Race: Black and White Boundaries*, Lamont, M. (ed). Chicago, University of Chicago Press: 371–90.

Goldberg, D.T. (1997) *Racial Subjects: Writing on Race in America*, New York: Routledge.

——(2002) *The Racial State*, London: Blackwell.

Harris, D.R. and Sim, J.J. (2002) "Who is multiracial? Assessing the complexity of lived race", *American Sociological Review*, 67: 614–27.

Hollinger, D.A. (2005) "The one-drop rule and the one-hate rule", *Daedalus*, 134(1): 18–28.

Holloway, S.R., Wright, R., Ellis, M. and East, M. (2009) "Place, scale and the racial claims made for multiracial children in the 1990 US Census", *Ethnic and Racial Studies*, 32(3): 522–47.

Holloway, S.R., Wright, R. and Ellis, M. (2012) "The racially fragmented city? Neighborhood racial segregation and diversity jointly considered", *The Professional Geographer*, 64(1): 63–82.

Johnston, R., Michael, P. and Forrest, J. (2006) "Ethnic residential segregation and assimilation in British towns and cities: A comparison of those claiming single and dual ethnic identities", *Migration Letters*, 3(1): 11–30.

Khanna, N. (2010) "'If you're half black, you're just black': Reflected appraisals and the persistence of the one-drop rule", *Sociological Quarterly*, 51(1): 96–121.

Liebler, C.A. (2010) "Homelands and indigenous identities in a multiracial era", *Social Science Research*, 39: 596–609.

Lipsitz, G. (1998) *Possessive Investment in Whiteness*, Philadelphia, PA: Temple University Press.

Mahtani, M. (2002) "Tricking the border guards: Performing race", *Environment and Planning D: Society and Space*, 20(4): 425–40.

Martin, D.G. (2003) "Enacting neighborhood", *Urban Geography*, 24(5): 361–85.

Nobles, M. (2000) *Shades of Citizenship: Race and the Census in Modern Politics*, Palo Alto, CA: Stanford University Press.

Omi, M. and Winant, H. (1994) *Racial Formation in the United States: From the 1960s to the 1990s*, New York: Routledge.

Perlmann, J. and Waters, M. (2005) *The New Race Question: How the Census Counts Multiracial People*, New York: Russell Sage.

Rockquemore, K., Brunsma, D. and Delgado, D. (2009) "Racing to theory or retheorizing race? Understanding the struggle to build a multiracial identity theory", *Journal of Social Issues*, 65(1): 13–34.

Rodriguez, C. (2000) *Changing Race: Latinos, the Census, and the History of Ethnicity in the United States*, New York: New York University Press.

Roth, W. (2005) "The end of the one-drop rule? Labeling of multiracial children in black intermarriages", *Sociological Forum*, 20(1): 35–67.

Saulny, S. (2011) "Census data presents rise in multiracial population of youths", *New York Times*, 24 March 2011, accessed online 4/2/2011 at http://www.nytimes.com/2011/03/25/us/25race.html?scp=1&sq=multiracial%20children&st=cse.

Shih, M., Bonam, C., Sanchez, D. and Peck, C. (2007) "The social construction of race: Biracial identity and vulnerability to stereotypes", *Cultural Diversity and Ethnic Minority Psychology*, 13(2): 125–33.

Takaki, R. (1989) *Strangers From a Different Shore: A History of Asian Americans*, Boston: Little, Brown.

US Census Bureau (2011) "Overview of race and Hispanic origin: 2010", 2010 Census Briefs, report C2010BR-02. Washington, DC: US Government Printing Office.

US Office of Management and Budget (1997) "Revisions to the standards for the classification of data on race and ethnicity", *Federal Register* 62(210): 5871–90. Washington, DC: US Government Printing Office.

Williams, K.M. (2006) *Mark One or More: Civil Rights in Multiracial America*, Ann Arbor, MI: University of Michigan Press.

7 Finding value on a council estate

Voices of white mothers with mixed-race children in St Anns, Nottingham

Lisa McKenzie

Introduction

This chapter introduces the voices of a group of white working-class women living on a council estate (public housing) in the UK drawing on a research project I conducted between 2005 and 2009, which examined how this group of women find value for themselves and their families. All of the women are mothers and have mixed-race children. The women reside on the St Anns estate in Nottingham, an inner-city neighbourhood which has been subject to poor housing, poverty and unemployment for many generations (Coates and Silburn 1970; Johns 2002). The women who live on this estate often say they suffer from negative stereotypes and stigmatisation because of where they live, because they are working class and because they have mixed-race children.

It is an unfortunate truth that over recent years there has been an excessive amount of moral panic, fear and political gesturing regarding and aimed at a specific section of the British working class. Those who live in social housing, have irregular and poorly paid employment and subsequently rely upon welfare benefits are often referenced within the 'underclass' discourse (Welshman 2006; Levitas 2005). However this moral outrage has been particularly vengeful in relation to council estate residents and, more specifically, those mothers who live on them with their children. It seems that the political classes from all parties have agreed that our British council estates are severe social problems; as the Conservative Party – and now coalition government – constantly reminds us, Britain is broken and its council estates 'are broken ghettos' (Riddell 2010; West 2009; Duncan-Smith 2008).

There has been a particular preoccupation with the notion that there are 'broken families' which are specifically located on the many council estates in Britain and the names of some of these estates have become shorthand for expressing everything that is wrong and loathsome about British society (Rogaly and Taylor 2009; Skeggs 2004). The St Anns estate in Nottingham is an example of how stigmatised neighbourhoods and their residents have become inextricably linked: as many residents note, you do not simply reside within St Anns, you *are* St Anns. The women who have taken part in this research acknowledge the stigmatisation of 'being St Anns' but also acknowledge that they have, as one of them put it, 'other crosses to bear': they have had sexual relationships with black men, and their children are mixed race which, they say, further stigmatises them as 'rough and ready' outside of the estate. As Caballero and Edwards (2010) illustrate in their tracing of the pathology of racially mixed families and children over the last 50 years, these stigmatised notions of 'lone mothers' and especially white lone mothers with mixed-race children are not new in British society but have a long, pervasive history.

However, while the politicians debate and the media paint a bleakly homogenous landscape of social alienation and abandonment of hope in poorer neighbourhoods, or of segregated inner-city communities embattled and suffering at the hands of 'mass immigration', the people who live on this estate in Nottingham tell of a far more complexly textured life. They speak of adaptation, cooperation and a reflexive awareness of their lives. Their accounts are inflected with recognition of heterogeneity and a sense of positive as well as negative aspects of estate life.

Getting to know this estate and its residents may open up a window in understanding how specific neighbourhoods become de-valued, and how families become stigmatised. In this case in Nottingham, the de-valuing process and stigmatisation is specifically related to being council estate mothers and white women who have had sexual relationships with black men, but also have mixed-race children. Nevertheless, and without neglecting the often harsh social realities families who live in poor neighbourhoods face, the women have found value locally, from their relationships with the West Indian community, and from the local status of being mothers to mixed-race children.

The poorest and most stigmatised neighbourhoods have little institutional capital, that is, employment, skills and education. These are the very resources that Pierre Bourdieu *et al.* (1999) argue allow groups, individuals and communities a status 'of value'. Those communities who are denied access to these valuable resources do not simply sit down and accept their fate, but instead engage in a local system that finds value for themselves and their families in local networks and a shared cultural understanding of how the estate works. The women in Nottingham who have taken part in this study invest within this local value system, and look to the resources within to feel valued and valuable, even when those local resources are often mis-recognised, dis-respected or are simply invisible to 'others'. This chapter explores the consequences of living on a council estate and becoming de-valued, thus raising important questions about class and race in Britain, the consequences of becoming stigmatised, and how communities, families and individuals manage the problems which arise through living in a poor neighbourhood and the ensuing stigmatisation.

The study

The St Anns estate is one of the poorest 10 per cent of neighbourhoods in the UK, and has been identified officially as 'socially excluded' (ONS 2007). Over decades, the neighbourhood has been subject to a number of harsh social realities: unemployment and low pay, and the lack of decent housing and good education (Johns 2002; Coates and Silburn 1970). Locally, it has become stigmatised with a reputation as a place to avoid, supposedly full of crime and drugs, single mums and benefit claimants. The neighbourhood also has a long history as the place where the poorest and migrant workers have resided in Nottingham; people from Ireland, the West Indies, Italy, Poland and South East Asia have been documented as living in St Anns since the early 1950s (Coates and Silburn 1970; Solomos 2003; Johns 2002). The neighbourhood has always been in flux, with people moving in and then, as they become more financially secure, often moving out. However the West Indian and especially Jamaican populations who arrived from the 1950s have stayed constant, creating homes, families and communities.

The research focused upon a group of 35 women who are white and are mothers to mixed-race children living on the St Anns council estate in Nottingham. The study aimed to examine how this group of women find value for themselves and their families when their estate and its residents are often represented as spaces and people of no or little value. The women varied in ages, with the youngest a 19-year-old mother with a six-week-old daughter, and the eldest a 56-year-old mother with eight children and numerous grandchildren and great-grandchildren. All of the children's fathers were African-Caribbean or of African-Caribbean descent, usually second or third generation migrant families predominantly coming from Jamaica in the late 1950s and early 1960s. The women referred to themselves as 'white English, Irish or Scottish'. They preferred to call their children 'mixed race' rather than 'dual heritage' which they thought sounded 'too American', and the women with older children said they were 'tired of it' (the description of their children) being changed every few years. Furthermore, they also objected to 'dual heritage' because it had become the preferred term used by the teachers at the local schools, and the women felt that neither they nor their children had been consulted by anyone in authority over which terms to use to describe them.

It is important that I discuss my own connection to the neighbourhood. As Minelle Mahtani discusses in this volume, all researchers are positioned in relation to their research subjects in some way, and it is important to interrogate this. I undertook the research, mapped the neighbourhood and interpreted the findings, but at the same time I am also a long-term resident of this estate, living in St Anns for more than 20 years with my own family. Therefore the ethnographic methodology used for the study did not present the usual challenges of access and familiarity: I was already part of the local community, my own children had attended the local schools and youth clubs and, as a white working-class woman and mother of mixed-race children who also had only lived on council estates, there was a commonality between the women and myself. Nevertheless, it would be wrong to underestimate not only the ease but also the difficulties within the relationships I formed with the women and their families. At times my positioning as resident and researcher was extremely strained; the unfair and negative representations of the women in this community often left them very defensive and since I also lived there, the women knew that I was aware of the stereotypes about the neighbourhood. Consequently there were initial concerns about how I might use my local knowledge and whether it would add to the negative portrayal of the estate and their families. The insider status I held was often difficult to negotiate within the research process and I cannot deny that my own position swings – from valueless St Anns resident to valuable academic researcher – have often left me feeling homeless.

Unfair representation and stigmatisation

Biased and mean representations of poor working-class people and the places where they live are widespread in the UK and have been well documented in the work of Skeggs (1997, 2004, 2009), Nayak (2009), Lawler (2008), Reay (2004), Haylett (2000, 2001, 2003), Munt (2000) and Sibley (1995). Lawler (2008: 133) argues that working-class people are rarely named as class subjects but are often known and reproduced as 'disgusting subjects', usually through descriptions of bodies and clothing, which are used as shorthand for stereotyping and identifying those who live on council estates. Skeggs (1997, 2004) shows in her work that working-class women in particular are subjects of ridicule and prurient fascination, often sexualised, and associated with dirt and disease. The contemporary representations that ridicule working-class women, and especially council estate mothers, relate to the wearing of track suits and gold jewellery, and having mixed-race babies – such portrayals are common within British television soap operas and comedy shows (e.g. Vicky Pollard in *Little Britain*, Bianca Butcher in *EastEnders*, Chantelle Garvey in *Benidorm*). These types of cultural reference can invoke signifiers that do a great deal of work in coding a way of life which has been deemed valueless, and become more poignant when we are discussing working-class women whose bodies, appearance, bearing and adornment are also central in coding working-class people. When those symbols are connected to living space – and in particular the term 'council estate' – it leaves the reader or the viewer to 'join up the dots of pathologisation' in order to see and understand the picture: that certain ways of dressing, speaking and also where you live indicate a despised 'class position but also an underlying pathology' (Lawler 2008: 133; Skeggs 2004: 37).

These representations of white working-class women have been documented previously. Bev Skeggs argues that working-class women are known as 'unrespectable' and have to work hard in becoming respectable usually through adopting middle-class practices, and by 'dis-identifying' from being working class (1997: 76–81). Chris Haylett further argues that to be 'white and working class' has become increasingly coded as 'backward' and un-modern (2001: 360–63). When negative representations of groups in society are commonplace it has an effect upon how those groups are understood and also how they understand themselves (Lawler 2008; Welshman 2006; Skeggs 1997, 2004; Haylett 2000, 2001). The women who live on the St Anns estate in Nottingham know what 'others' think of them and a common theme in their interviews is the notion of being demeaned, 'looked down on' and made to 'feel small', as discussed in the next section.

Being looked down on

The women had an acute understanding of how they were known and 'looked down on' in wider Nottingham and society generally because they lived on a council estate. They never denied where they thought they were positioned, often saying we are 'at the bottom', or 'lower class'. Yet they never tried to identify with 'middle-class culture' in order to become 'respectable', instead finding value for themselves and their children from within the community, and through engaging in a local culture they described as 'being St Anns'. This was a local identity which was valued and had meaning for the women within the estate, but was not necessarily a valued identity that might be universally understood, such as the middle-class, educated and respectable identity that Bev Skeggs (1997) notes.

The women discussed at great length the ways they were represented in the media. For example, Tanya, a 27-year-old mother with three children under the age of five, explained that she could not understand why she had noticed 'on the telly' that when a woman was supposed to be 'common' (Matt Lucas's Vicky Pollard, Catherine Tate's Lauren, and Bianca from *EastEnders* were mentioned) they wore big hooped gold earrings, which she liked and she thought they suited her. Zena, another mum living on the estate with her two-year-old son and 12-year-old daughter, told me that she 'knew' that some people would call her a chav not only because she liked wearing a lot of gold jewellery but also because of the ethnicity of her children: 'too much gold, tracksuit and trainers, black baby in the pram'.

Gina was 21, pregnant and lived alone with her six-month-old and two-year-old sons who she described as 'quarter caste' – their father was mixed race and lived on the estate with his mother, who was also involved in this research. Gina was one of many of the mothers who told me she felt an acute stigma, particularly whenever she went to any of the benefit agencies. Although Gina was studying at a local college she claimed income support and housing benefit, and therefore was in constant contact with 'officials'. Gina told me that every time she gave her address to any of the 'officials' there was often a silence as they mentally processed her single-parent status, the ethnicity of her children, and then her address in St Anns: 'I know what they're thinking you can see it ticking over in their brain as you wait for them to think "oh it's one of them from there"'. Although negative social assumptions relating to lone mothers, or mothers who live on council estates have been noted previously (Skeggs 1997; Lawler 2000; Gillies 2007) the women in St Anns are particularly sensitive not only to the negative assumptions relating to being a lone mother living on a council estate, but also and in particular to being a white mother to mixed-race children. All of the women talked to me about how they were often sexualised because their children were signifiers and ultimate proof that they had sexual relationships with black men. Zena said to me that everyone thinks 'she's up for it', and Lynn, a woman in her 40s with an adult daughter, described being known as 'rough' because she came from a council estate, but also 'ready' meaning sexually available.

The women described their feelings of 'being looked down on' usually through their contact with 'others' who did not live on the estate. They also recognised the many aspects of their lives which stigmatised them. Mandy had lived in St Anns with her own family her whole life and now she was in her mid-30s and a mother she lived with her three sons on the estate. Mandy's middle son is autistic and she was advised by a social worker to go to the Gingerbread club, a local group of Nottingham mothers who met up with their disabled children. Mandy felt awkward when she arrived, because the women there were 'not like' her:

> Well I thought the people were posh people do you know what I mean the way they looked at me I felt really small I had to come out and my kids were playing up basically but I felt they were looking at me cos I was white and they [my kids] were mixed race. … no one talked to me yeah I felt that if I had said well … if they had said where are you from and I'd had said I'm from St Anns they would have said oh yeah I can see why, that is how I felt … I wont there very long at all they dint mek me feel welcome. That Gingerbread club has been around for years I don't know if it's still going and I think that was one of the things that made me feel more secluded with my disabled son cos I felt like people were looking at me all the time at that Gingerbread club there was a lot of people there with disabled children do you know what I mean but they seemed posh and I felt that I was lower class.

Mandy was only one of the many women who told me about their experiences of feeling stigmatised, and 'looked down on'. As a result, they were extremely reluctant to meet anyone who they thought might be 'posh' or might not understand their lives and, consequently, demean them. The women in St Anns did not appear to engage in finding value in a 'respectable performance' as Skeggs notes (1997: 94), rather, they looked for value, and resources of value, from what was available to them. This meant that some of the heavily stereotyped and negative aspects about 'being St Anns' were celebrated by the women. All of them challenged the 'others' who looked down on them, stating that 'they could not live one day in our lives'. Furthermore, they also took pride in the fact that they 'badded it out' on the estate, finding a sense of value from overcoming the difficulties they experienced. The women whom I met faced the challenges of living on the estate, and because of this valued 'being St Anns'; meeting those challenges and dealing with the difficulties that the estate brought allowed the women to talk proudly about their daily lives. Therefore it is important to understand what 'being St Anns' means, as it is an identity which is recognised as of value within the neighbourhood and to the women.

'Being St Anns': the 'Jamaicanization' of a neighbourhood

'Being St Anns' was the way most women I spoke to described themselves. 'I'm typical St Anns' or 'when you're St Anns' was how the women often started a conversation. Being connected to the neighbourhood was extremely important – in order to show they were St Anns, the women described their family connections in great detail, the length of time they had lived in the neighbourhood and the depth of local knowledge they held about the area and its residents. This network and engagement located in the neighbourhood culture also meant that you could easily be recognised through ways of dressing and speaking as well as through your 'taste' in music, food and social events. As noted above, most of the women wore a lot of gold jewellery, such as big creole earrings, some had gold capped teeth, and expensive and branded sportswear and trainers were important for themselves and their children. These were ways that the women could show that they belonged to the estate; they knew what was valued, and ensured that their children were also valued. The women discussed the ways and methods they might save or earn money in order to buy expensive and designer label clothes for their children. Birthday parties and christenings were also very popular on the estate and were events where the women 'showed off' their children. These gatherings were lavish affairs with expensive birthday cakes and gifts of jewellery, as well as new and extensively planned outfits for mothers and children.

'Being St Anns' was also related to how you spoke in addition to how you looked and dressed. The distinct St Anns dialect – a mixture of the local Nottingham accent interspersed with Jamaican words and speech patterns – was described by some of the women as the 'street' language of St Anns. I met two sisters, 'Kirsty' and 'Lucy', who were in their late teens and both of whose 'baby fathers' (a term used by the West Indian community to mean a child's biological father) came from Jamaica. They had lived on the estate since leaving Glasgow with their parents as very young children.

LUCY: People has said to me 'you think you're black cos you talk like that' well actually no I don't, I see it as street even now I'd get it as a big woman (adult) in the pub you know people say why you speak like that and I'm well 'that's how I've always spoke'.

KIRSTY: Well a lot of people have said that I think I'm black and I wanna be black but I don't see it like that I see it like it was the community I was brought up in you know if you stick a black person in a white community they're gonna grow up white and if you stick a white person in a black community they're obviously gonna have black ways about them.

Although the use of specific West Indian styles of speaking and dressing are valued on the estate, these are not the only sites of value relating to the West Indian community: the Jamaican families in particular are themselves valued within the community. Therefore being a part of one of the Jamaican families holds considerable worth. Many of the women discussed this as being particularly significant to 'being St Anns' and the value of this specific multi-cultural identity has been described by the women as a 'modern', urban identity. The women on the estate understood that to be white and working class has become a de-valued position over the last 30 years: cultureless, backward and un-modern (Haylett 2003: 333). They recognised this through valuing what they thought was 'black culture' in contrast to what they described as being 'white'.

Once you go black you never go back

The ways in which heavily stereotyped images of black masculinity centring about sexual potency, 'coolness', criminality and macho aggression have both emerged and infiltrated the British psyche in recent years, especially in relation to white working-class youth culture, have been well mapped by various scholars (Hebdige 1979; Hewitt 1986; Back 1996; Gilroy 2000). The valued understanding of 'blackness' and Jamaican culture in St Anns is equated with such ideas about black West Indian masculinity and is recognised as extremely prestigious in and around the estate. As such, you do not necessarily have to be 'black' or male in order to benefit from its value as this masculinity is strongly associated with a street and urban culture and is expressed through language, music, food and dress.

Les Back notes that the histories and cultural politics of the Caribbean and black America have formed the raw materials for a creative process in which 'black culture is actively made and re-made' (1996: 184). Based on his research during the 1990s in South London he argues that a constant process of 'fashioning and re-fashioning' is happening within distinct and particular urban social relations, creating a cultural hybridity (ibid.). St Anns in Nottingham has all the elements in place for the creative processes that allow 'black culture to be re-made' in negotiation with white working-class residents (ibid.). This is an extremely interesting and relevant use of 'cultural hybridity' (Bhabha 1990) which has emerged in St Anns. It adds another dimension in understanding contemporary identities and theorising possible fragmentation in white working-class understandings of themselves especially within multi-cultural urban neighbourhoods. It is not only the white mothers with mixed-race children who engage in this hybrid and entwined culture of 'blackness' and 'working-classness' – such behaviour is widely understood and practised throughout the estate. Claire, a mother with a 10-year-old daughter who describes herself as 'a lifer in St Anns', explained how this particular understanding of 'blackness' works in practice:

> You see these white guys trying to walk like black people and you think God it must take you all day to get across the street but you're prepared to do it to keep this image and they have this tough face and you think 'you're not black'.

This is only one of many observations by the women in this research of how 'blackness' is often demonstrated within the estate, especially by young white men who appear to have practised 'being authentic' within the community through the visual markers of ways of dressing, walking and speaking. In fact many of the women struggled to explain their own 'feelings' of ethnicity and the impact 'mixedness' had upon the estate and their own lives. Gina, who had previously complained about how she thought the agencies see her, then went on to discuss how she sees herself:

> I don't see myself as full white neither do my friends especially black friends I don't think they see me as white or a white person, they know I'm white but they look at you different you know cos you've got mixed-race kids.

Gina also extended this complexity to her personal relationships:

> Yeah I have tried to go out with a white boy before but the white boys think they're black they've got gold teeth they've got the black image so you might as well go out with someone real.

When Gina talks about 'someone real' she is talking about 'authenticity' on the estate, and what is real and authentic for Gina is the black male, who also holds the most value for her. She demonstrates this in this next extract, in talking about how she thinks about 'white men':

> It might seem horrible but you know I think boring old white pub man, and I think of my Dad who just plays football and I know black people play football you know but I just think like beer belly and how they dress and then black people it is different you know you can go to all these different dances, different music, food and it's interesting.

It seems that the taking on of 'black traditions and style' has resulted in a radical reconfiguration of white working-class culture in multi-ethnic locales (Gilroy 2004; Back and Ware 2002; Hewitt 1986). This has led Gilroy to suggest that 'Black culture has become a class culture … as two generations have appropriated it and discovered its seductive meaning for their own' (2000: 273). The women in St Anns understand the value and worth of what Gilroy terms 'black culture' and have appropriated it into their own lives, passing it down to their children. In their interviews, they discuss how 'mixing' their own white working-class culture with an African-Caribbean culture has created something in the community that is superior to what they call 'the old days', when everything was 'white and boring'. The women on this estate constantly talk of the pride they have of being 'more than just white' and of their 'beautiful mixed-race children' along with their modern 'multi-cultural families'. They regarded this mixing as the positive side of their physical, social and class positions – which without exception they understood as being 'at the bottom'. It was this part of their lives that they were most proud of, and this was apparent in the way in which they talked about their children as being special and beautiful. Moreover, they thought that they had given their children something which they and the estate valued: a birth status 'of not being just white'.

All of the women discussed how important this sharing of culture had been and the impact it had made on their lives. Della, who was 38 and raising her five children alone, told me that being part of the black British and Jamaican community in St Anns and engaging in the culture connected with this community was extremely important for her. This was not just because she had mixed-race children:

> I've never really mixed with white people to me to go to a white club to me I don't feel like I fit in, if I go to a black club I feel more comfortable because that's the kind of music I like. ... I was into it even before I met the kids' dad. ... I always mixed with black people so as I say for me to go to a white club I can't go to it cos I'm not into that sort of music I feel like the people aren't the same as me even though they're the same colour as me ... you know people will say to me do you know you're white I know I'm white but it's hard to explain to someone who don't get it.

Lorraine, also in her 30s, was another single mother with five children and, like many of the mothers, had lived on the estate for most of her life and felt she had a connection with the Jamaican community. Lorraine's family had moved into the estate in the early 1970s when they first arrived in Nottingham from Ireland. She was proud of her connection with the Jamaican community in St Anns and talked about her childhood memories of dancing to reggae music and eating Jamaican food. Now Lorraine has her own children she feels that it is important to cook Jamaican food at home. She also told me that there is a value attached to how authentically you can make Jamaican food, which is part of a wider value system of knowledge about Jamaican culture. Lorraine told me that anyone can cook chicken, but asked how many women her age, white or black, can cook good green banana:

> Well I think Irish and black mix really well they just do back in the day what was it no blacks, no dogs, no Irish what can you say ... my auntie always went out with black guys so I used to go round there and she used to cook and the music was there so I was into it from about 10 ... I like the reggae music and the Jamaican food true dat I only listen to bare

> reggae music now and every day I have to cook bare food I have to cook curries, rice, yam, green banana I have to cook everything how much white woman can cook all dem tings.

Appropriating the local culture, and engaging in the local value system through what you wear, eat and how you speak, as Butler argues (2006), is a matter of embodied social practice, a constant reiteration and 'performance' of particular discourses. The particular discourse here is of people who have become known as 'socially excluded', outside the norms of society. Haylett (2001: 353) and Skeggs (2004: 111) argue that there has been a racialisation of a specific group of white working-class people as 'the dirty white'. This group understand who they are and their own social positions through how they are judged and stigmatised in the media and wider social discourse. On this basis, it becomes all the more important for the women living in St Anns to 'feel comfortable and fit in' within the estate which, simultaneously, allows them to be easily recognised on the outside.

'Out of many comes one people'

In St Anns, the embodied and cultural practices described above and the dialogue of recognition on the estate determines how 'authentic' you are. All of the women I spoke to recognised these practices and engaged in them, regardless of their age. This type of street culture generally is associated with young people and youth, but on the estate it is associated with 'being local' and 'being St Anns'. Dawn, who was 32 and had three children, of which the eldest two were white, told me that:

> Well you have to fit you have to fit like … I've been here all my life it's funny really cos when I go out cos most of my friends are either black or mixed race I think I've probably only got three or four white people who are my friends … and for instance I was out a couple of months ago with a white friend and we went to a pub where she likes to go and it was a white pub and I felt uncomfortable.

Dawn went on to say where she did feel comfortable, which she described as 'black places':

> I feel like I fit in that kind of place I feel like I slip in a lot better I love the music that's my music … I play the music for all three of my kids and my daughter she's white and she understands patois and sings to all the words.

This connection to what they call 'black culture', and the 'black community' is important to the women as it is through this engagement that they feel like people of value on the estate. Nevertheless, there is often another aspect to this connection. When the women spoke of the things they liked about St Anns, the area's multi-culturalism was something they often brought up. Sharon, a woman in her 50s, has eight children of whom the six eldest are white with mixed-race children – including Tanya, discussed earlier – and the two youngest are mixed race. In talking of all the things they liked about St Anns, Tanya and Sharon highlighted the local schools. Like many of the women, they held the primary schools in high regard and told me they believed their children were getting something really important by going to school in St Anns. The 'multi-culturalism' of the schools was often brought up as the extra value that their children were gaining:

TANYA: That's one of the positive things about St Anns for the fact is that if you go to certain areas where the kids are all white then them kids have a thing there like a barrier with them people … cos they haven't mixed with them when they've mixed and they're all multi-cultural and they have had to learn things and then even in the classrooms here in St Anns the teachers teach them what comes from the Chinese people and whatever else there is round here and that's good our kids don't grow up ignorant they know about multi-cultural things and that's good.

SHARON: I think that Sycamore is a good school they do loads of things for multi-cultural things … yeah they need to know about all different cultures the white and the black culture that's what I think is important both.

TANYA: I believe that there should be more multi-cultural teaching cos it's alright having them all together and them not learning from each other I think it should be a topic at all schools like Art, Maths and English yes because this is a multi-cultural country now.

SHARON: Well I think that eventually this country will be mixed race cos there's that many black and white people going together there's a lot of mixed race cos it's not the richer ones that are mixing it's us the lower ones so maybe our class will not be white anymore we will end up mixed race well that means that life's more interesting for us cos life was boring when I was young I've found out that it's more interesting being with a black man put it this way I've done more since I've been with them and I've learnt more and seen more than when I was with a white man.

Although it has often been argued that multi-culturalism is a vague and confused concept having different meanings to different people (Modood 2004), the people in St Anns explained their relationships, families and community as multi-cultural, and understood it as a sharing of culture, 'mixing it up'. The women often used the Jamaican national statement, 'out of many comes one people', as a way to explain what St Anns has within its boundaries, and how it should be viewed. One community, many differences, but ultimately 'being St Anns' and having this shared understanding is important.

Sharon's personal understanding of multi-culturalism and mixedness has a much wider relevance. She describes herself as white and working class; she worked in the textile factories in Nottingham before de-industrialisation hit the city. Sharon had six children from her previous relationship with her white working-class husband. However she told me that being with her black partner meant that life was more 'interesting' now, and had given her a value within the estate that she had not experienced previously: 'you used to go to parties and there was boring food but now it's all different food different music yeah I am proud of my mixed relationship'. Like all of the women on the estate, Sharon was extremely proud of her mixed-race family, and the thought of the white working class no longer being white was not a worrying prospect for her. In actual fact, many of the women on the estate thought that all this mixing 'is good for us'.

Conclusion

Within this chapter I have discussed how the women with mixed-race children living on the St Anns estate that I spoke to find value. The ways in which they do this are particularly important in light of their feelings of being de-valued by those who 'look down' on them, ridicule who they are, and stigmatise their lives and ways of being. The women have very little of the institutional capital which Bourdieu (1986) says is needed to be a person of value: they have limited formal education, those who work tend to be in unskilled and low-paid jobs, and they and their families live on a council estate. Being a person of value is as important here as it is in any group within society. However the women believe they have been socially rejected by those on the 'outside', and compensate by engaging in what is local, available and, importantly, demonstrable. This local practice forms an autonomous entity which is defined by a negative polarisation to the norms of wider society and creates an alternative value system. By creating an alternative value system, those who are marginalised can create feelings of worth, power and status on the inside of their neighbourhood and amongst those who recognise and take part in the alternative value system (Cohen 2002: 28). Due to the complex nature of the estate, the alternative value system, and the elements which make up this system, are difficult to pin down. But the system also takes different forms for the different groups within it. For women, a high value is placed on motherhood and therefore being a mother ranks highly on the estate. Indeed, being a mother and coping with the difficulties of living on the estate are often the only things the women cite as being proud of in their lives.

There is a real and acknowledged value in engaging in the local culture which has been heavily influenced by black Jamaican culture, particularly for the mothers who have mixed-race children. Being authentic to the neighbourhood, being known and fitting in are other elements in becoming a person of value on the estate, but also to whom and how you are connected is equally important. In particular, there has been an exchange of culture on this estate: the women who live here are extremely proud of their success in 'mixing'. While this type of 'cultural mixing' has often been associated with 'youth culture', in St Anns in Nottingham it is not limited to young people only; it has become a hybrid and interchangeable culture that has grown throughout the whole community over a 50 year period of the West Indian and white working-class communities living side by side.

Other literature relating to mixed families often focuses upon the negatives, the difficulties of inter-racial relationships and mixed identities. Vicki Harman's (2010) study and Ravinder Barn's (1999) work relating to social work practice highlight how white mothers with mixed-race children are often isolated and subject to racism with little support, thus urging professionals to consider the specific difficulties mixed families encounter. Meanwhile, France Winddance Twine's study of mixed families in the UK focuses on how white parents to what she calls 'children of black Caribbean ancestry' (2010: 880) negotiate racism and teach their children 'racial literacy' through engaging in black cultural forms.

However this study with white mothers in St Anns shows a much more complex picture of modern British life, especially for those who live in the most disadvantaged neighbourhoods where there has been a long history of migration. The women on this estate have a high regard for the community where they live, recognising the local support systems which can have huge benefits for families living on the estate, as well as penalties for the mothers in wider society. The women in St Anns also value the Jamaican community and engage and invest in Jamaican culture, through food, music, clothing and ways of speaking. Twine also notes that white parents with mixed-race children invest in black cultural forms, but as ways of teaching their children how to cope with racism and their blackness. The women in St Anns do not invest in these cultural forms as ways of teaching racial literacy to their children but because it has a value on the estate and adds value to the women who have become de-valued by the inter-sectionality between their whiteness and working-classness. This picture of modern Britain is complex. It shows how identity and community are closely linked, especially in stigmatised working-class neighbourhoods. The dynamic nature of multi-cultural Britain, and how racial identities are much more fluid than one may imagine, means that mixing on this estate is highly valued. It offers status and an opportunity to be more than a working-class white woman alongside a chance to engage in a contemporary multi-cultural Britain that in many other ways excludes and stigmatises this group of women.

References

Back, L. (1996) *New Ethnicities and Urban Culture: Racisms and Multi-Culture in Young Lives*, London: Routledge.

Back, L. and Ware, V. (2002) *Out of Whiteness: Colour, Politics and Culture*, Chicago: University of Chicago Press.

Barn, R. (1999) 'White mothers, mixed-parentage children and child welfare', *British Journal of Social Work* 29(2): 269–84.

Bhabha, H. (1990) *Nation and Narration*, London: Routledge.
Bourdieu, P. (1977) *Outline of a Theory of Practice*, Cambridge: Cambridge University Press.
——(1986) *Distinction: A Critique of the Social Judgement of Taste*, London: Routledge.
——(1990) *The Logic of Practice*, Cambridge: Polity Press.
Bourdieu, P., Accardo, A., Balazs, G., Beaude, S., Bonvin, F., Bourdieu, E. Borgois, P., Brocolichi, S., Champagne, P., Christin, R., Faguer, J., Garcia, S., Lenoir, R., Euvrard, F., Pialoux, M., Pinto, L., Podalydes, D., Sayad, A., Soclic, C. and Wacquant, C. (1999) *The Weight of the World: Social Suffering in Contemporary Society*, Cambridge: Polity Press.
Butler, J. (2006) *Gender Trouble: Feminism and the Subversion of Identity*, London: Routledge.
Caballero, C. and Edwards, R. (2010) *Lone Mothers of Mixed Racial and Ethnic Children: Then and Now*, London: Runnymede Trust.
Coates, K. and Silburn, R. (1970) *Poverty the Forgotten Englishman*, London: Penguin Books.
Cohen, S. (2002) *Folk Devils and Moral Panics: 30th Anniversary Edition: Creation of Mods and Rockers*, London: Routledge.
Duncan-Smith, I. (2008) 'Broken ghettos', *The Times*, 30 November: 1–2.
Gillies, V. (2007) *Marginalised Mothers: Exploring Working-Class Experiences of Parenting*, London: Routledge.
Gilroy, P. (2000) *There Ain't No Black in the Union Jack*, London: Routledge.
——(2004) *After Empire: Multiculture or Postcolonial Melancholia*, London: Routledge.
Harman, V. (2010) 'Social work practice and lone mothers of mixed-parentage children', *British Journal of Social Work* 40: 391–406.
Haylett, C. (2000) 'Modernisation, welfare and "third way" politics: limits to theorising in "thirds"?', *Transactions of the Institute of British Geographers* 26 (1): 43–56.
——(2001) 'Illegitimate subjects? Abject whites, neo-liberal modernisation and middle-class multiculturalism', *Environment and Planning D: Society and Space* 19 (3): 351–70.
——(2003) *Culture, Class and Urban Policy: Reconsidering Inequality*, Oxford: Blackwell Publishing.
Hebdige, D. (1979) *Subculture: The Meaning of Style*, London: Methuen.
Hewitt, R. (1986) *White Talk, Black Talk: Inter-Racial Friendship and Communication amongst Adolescents*, Cambridge: Cambridge University Press.
Johns, R. (2002) *St Anns: Inner City Voices*, Warwick: Plowright Press.
Lawler, S. (2000) *Mothering the Self: Mothers, Daughters, Subjects*, London: Routledge.
——(2004) 'Rules of engagement: habitus, power and resistance' in Adkins, L. and Skeggs, B. (eds), *Feminism After Bourdieu*, Oxford: Blackwell Publishing.
——(2005) 'Disgusted subjects: the making of middle-class identities', *The Sociological Review* 53 (3): 429–46.
——(2008) *Identity; Sociological Perspectives*, Cambridge: Polity Press.
Levitas, R. (2005 [1999]) *The Inclusive Society*, London: Macmillan.
Modood, T. (2004) 'Capitals, ethnic identity and educational qualifications', *Cultural Trends* 13 (2): 87–105.
Munt, S. (ed.) (2000) *Cultural Studies and the Working Class: Subject to Change*, London: Cassell.
Nayak, A. (2006) 'Displaced masculinities: chavs, youth and class in the post-industrial city', *Sociology* 40 (5): 813–31.

——(2009) 'Beyond the pale: chavs, youth and social class' in Sveinsson, K. (ed.) *Who Cares about the White Working Class*?, London: Runnymede Trust.

ONS (Office for National Statistics) (2007) *The English Indices of Deprivation 2007*, London: HMSO Communities and Local Government Publication.

Reay, D. (2004) 'Gendering Bourdieu's concept of capitals? Emotional capital, women and social class' in Adkins, L. and Skeggs, B. (eds) *Feminism after Bourdieu*, Oxford: Blackwell.

Reay, D. and Lucey, H. (2000) '"I don't really like it here but I don't want to be anywhere else": children and inner city council estates', *Antipode* 32 (4): 410–28.

Riddell, P. (2010) 'We're living in broken Britain, say most voters', *The Times*, 9 February: 9–10.

Rogaly, B. and Taylor, B. (2009) *Moving Histories of Class and Community*, London: Palgrave Macmillan.

Sibley, D. (1995) *Geographies of Exclusion: Society and Difference in the West*, London: Routledge.

Skeggs, B. (1997) *Formations of Class and Gender*, London: Routledge.

——(2004) *Class, Self and Culture*, London: Routledge.

——(2005) 'The re-branding of class: propertising culture', in Devine F., Savage M., Scott J. and Crompton, R. (eds) *Rethinking Class: Cultures, Identities and Lifestyles*, Basingstoke: Palgrave.

——(2009) 'Haunted by the spectre of judgment: respectability, value and affect in class relations', in Sveinsson, K. (ed.) *Who Cares about the White Working Class*, London: Runnymede Trust.

Solomos, J. (2003, 3rd edn) *Race and Racism in Britain*, Basingstoke: Palgrave.

Twine, F. W. (2010) *A White Side of Black Britain: The Concept of Racial Literacy*, Durham, NC: Duke University Press.

Welshman, J. (2006) *Underclass: A History of the Excluded 1880–2000*, London: Hambledon Continuum.

West, E. (2009) 'How to create an underclass: stalk council estates handing out condoms', the *Telegraph*, 14 August 2009: 18.

8 A descriptive account of those self-identifying as of mixed ethnicity in Great Britain

Lucinda Platt

Background

The presence of those designated as being of mixed ethnicity has been a source of celebration and anxiety across countries. Nowhere is this more evident than in Great Britain where the last decade, since mixed-group categories were first included in the national Censuses, has seen a proliferation of interest in the implications for conceptions of ethnicity and 'race' and understandings of social stratification, social interaction and national identity. There has been increasing media as well as academic attention paid to the 'mixed' population of Great Britain, supported by claims that it is the 'fastest growing minority group' (Phillips 2009; see also Rees *et al.* 2010: ix, 2011). Its growth and apparent visibility is used as a means of marking the changing and developing composition of British society.

Yet, while claims to the significance of increases in the mixed ethnicity populations abound in popular discourse, and estimates of the extent and growth of the population have been substantially refined, current quantitative analysis is largely descriptive (see e.g. Platt 2009). Theoretical framing and analysis of determinants draws explicitly or implicitly on the much more extensive US literature. The extent to which such perspectives are an adequate representation of the British case have only begun to be directly interrogated (Muttarak and Heath 2010; Model and Fisher 2002), yet there may be a range of reasons why the British case may be distinctive, given the UK's very particular history of migration and settlement of minority groups, the relationship with former colonies, and the complex interplay of exclusionary and inclusionary policies (Model and Fisher 2002; Joppke 1999).

Thus, while understanding the overarching literature on the ways in which interethnic unions are formed and the interpretation of their implications can contribute to claims to celebrate the growth of 'mixedness' in Great Britain, it is unlikely to provide the whole story. Moreover, it needs to be supplemented by analysis of the experience of the children of such unions, that is those who either designate themselves as 'mixed' or who have parents from different ethnic groups (typically the majority and a minority group).

The traditional approach has regarded interethnic partnerships as marking the 'last and most critical step' (Wildsmith *et al.* 2003: 565) in an overarching process of immigrant or minority group assimilation (Duncan and Lieberson 1959). From this perspective, the prevalence and increase in interethnic partnerships act as a 'benchmark for race relations' (Fryer 2007: 73), thus representing an open and integrated society. If those from different backgrounds chose each other in the context of the most intimate of relations, then that implied that the 'melting pot' had been achieved. Similarly, evidence of substantial proportions in the population of mixed heritage or ethnicity, typically the outcome of such partnerships in the same country, is often taken to evidence the openness of society and the success of the multicultural project. A monocultural society cannot then be maintained in the face of the diverse social relations of its population, and the potential and willingness of that population to acknowledge its various antecedents.

In such multicultural success models social and economic 'assimilation' are often elided, with marital assimilation apparently presupposing economic assimilation (Gordon 1964; see also Hwang *et al.* 1997; Meng and Gregory 2005). However, whether that is in fact the reality is contested (Song 2009). There is substantial research demonstrating that minority group members who marry majority group members tend to be more highly educated (Kalmijn and van Tubergen 2006), but this is not the same as arguing that in aggregate increasing rates of interethnic marriage indicate increasing economic equality. The parents of the mixed ethnicity population may be distinctive in a range of ways (Kantarevic 2004; Duncan and Trejo 2007; Furtado 2006); and access to majority resources (or equal resources from both sides of the multiple heritage) does not necessarily follow from parentage. By contrast with Furtado, van Ours and Veenman (2008) have suggested that having a majority group mother can favour children's educational outcomes – in the specific case of Moluccan–Dutch partnerships. The authors warn against generalising their finding; and given the significance of national context and composition, it is particularly hard to extrapolate from such findings to another country. At the same time, in the UK there has been some indication from research in specific fields that those of mixed ethnicity may face specific disadvantages, rather than the ability to capitalise on potential sources of advantage offered by multiple heritages (Barn *et al.* 2005; Barn and Harman 2006; see also the discussion in Edwards *et al.* 2010). Model and Fisher (2002) were agnostic about the implications of the greater openness of the UK relative to the US to interethnic marriages. But while there is an increasingly rich understanding of the identification of those of mixed or multiple heritage and their willingness to engage with those heritages, as well as of the diversity among them (Song 2010), we lack a simple overview of the experiences of the 'mixed' generations and how these relate to these differing expectations and claims.

It is important, also, to consider that claims about the significance of an acknowledged or increasing mixed ethnicity population are still typically premised on an essentialist approach to ethnicity; that is, the notion of groups mixing, which brings about such possibilities for bi- (or multi-) heritage categories. The suggestion that mixed ethnicities can themselves constitute a 'group' in their own right is also highly problematic. It implies that having parents of different ethnic groups is in itself sufficient to create a common bond, and thereby constitute a bounded ethnic group, between otherwise unlike individuals. However it is arguable whether claims for recognition of multiple heritage thereby create the conditions for construction of bounded ethnic identities across those of mixed ethnicity, either through the recognition of imagined common antecedents or for more instrumental purposes (Barth 1969; Weber 1978). Indeed it may more convincingly be argued that claims for recognition of mixedness are better understood as claims for singularity, albeit within the acknowledged social context of racialised relations (Edwards *et al.* 2010).

Patterns of mixed ethnicity that emerge in the data such as I describe below, are not a simple 'objective' description of those who have parents from different heritages, but reflect the choices people make when faced with a series of boxes within which to define themselves (Aspinall 2010), and the way these boxes themselves have been subject to negotiation and reformulation (Burton *et al.* 2010). Moreover, evidence from other countries suggests that choices about ethnicity may themselves reflect a number of considerations including both the context in which respondents are asked (Harris and Sim 2002), and the social location associated with particular ethnic groups (Duncan and Trejo 2007; Finnäs and O'Leary 2003).

Nevertheless it remains an empirical question the extent to which those who do engage in self-categorisation in terms of one of the mixed ethnicity categories reveal a distinctive profile, or to what extent they demonstrate a new generation of minority experience in which not only the fact of 'mixedness' but also their achievements and outcomes demonstrate declining ethnic stratification within British society. Conversely does a broad overview of the experience of mixed groups tend to locate them in a midway position between the experience of non-mixed minorities and majority? Or is there evidence that those of mixed heritage are in fact more marginalised, being placed in an ambiguous position in a society where racialised boundaries are highly significant? While it is beyond the scope of this chapter to properly test any of these claims, the overview of key characteristics and how they vary within mixed groups as well as between mixed and other ethnic categories in Britain, suggests that there may be no single answer: that it will depend on what is being investigated and a more detailed understanding of the circumstances surrounding the different ethnic groups. Overall the implication of this chapter's account is that promoting the growth of 'mixedness' as signifying that Britain has entered a post-racial era is perhaps premature.

Categorising mixed groups

The first time that the British census asked people to identify their ethnic group it did not include any mixed categories. Individuals were expected to find a place to fit them which by implication accorded them the position of their minority parent. There were criticisms and objections to this effective racialisation of those with multiple heritages (albeit the Census ethnic group categories were always implicitly intended to measure the 'non-White' population of the UK (Salt 1996; see also Ballard 1997)), and debates on how best to capture the diversity and change in the composition of the population (Aspinall 2000, 2003; Berthoud 1998). The result was the inclusion of four mixed ethnicity categories in the Census questionnaire for England and Wales, which have been retained in the 2011 categories and which have informed collection of ethnic group throughout government and research surveys. These categories are: White and Black Caribbean; White and Black African; White and Asian; and Other Mixed ethnic group. By offering a series of mixed ethnic group categories, the 2001 census and subsequent surveys have thereby encouraged respondents to consider their ethnicity in terms of heritage and relative to their parents' ethnic group(s).

The inclusion of mixed categories in the national classification of ethnic groups from 2001 onwards has provided the opportunity to consider at a population level and in much more detail than hitherto, the characteristics and experience of those of mixed ethnicity. The distinction of separate mixed categories also allows us to compare their experiences with those of the White majority, who typically (though not always) make up one side of the parentage of those of mixed ethnicity, as well as with those who identify with the minority groups that make up the other side of their heritage. That is, we can compare those who are White and Black Caribbean with those who are White and with those who are Black Caribbean; those who are White and Black African with those who are White and those who are Black African, and those who are White and Asian with those who are White and those who are Indian. While not all 'White and Asian' respondents have an Indian parent, the vast majority do, which makes this if not an exact comparison at least the most appropriate, especially given the very different experiences of the different South Asian groups. The remaining mixed ethnicity group, 'Other Mixed', incorporates all other forms of mixed or multiple heritage, including those of more than one minority heritage. However, since the classification aggregates all these, the group is not susceptible to distinct analysis. For the descriptions of the 'mixed' population as a whole all four groups are included together, while the follow-up analyses focus on the three distinct mixed groups. This potential for fine-grained comparison presented by this particular categorisation forms the basis for the descriptive analysis of the Labour Force Survey that follows.

Source data

The description of the demographics and characteristics of those of mixed ethnicity in Great Britain presented in this chapter derives from analysis of the Labour Force Survey (LFS). The LFS is a quarterly survey of private households that is intended to be representative of the UK population. There are around 50,000 responding households covered by the LFS in Great Britain (the focus of this study) each quarter.[1] Households are followed up for five consecutive quarters, and therefore only around a fifth of the sampled population is new to the survey at any quarter. To simplify the analysis such that it covers unique individuals only, I therefore retain only those in households which are newly included (i.e. are at their first interview wave). In Great Britain, those who classify themselves as belonging to one of the four mixed ethnicity categories in the standard classification form only very small proportions of the overall population. I therefore pool a large number of quarters to provide sufficient sample sizes for adequate description and analysis. Specifically, I pool the 28 quarters covering seven years from the last quarter of 2003 to the third quarter of 2010. This provides a dataset of 688,028 individuals of whom 6,949, or around 1 per cent, are from one of the four mixed ethnicity categories.

Overview of the mixed ethnic group population

Table 8.1 shows all the detailed ethnic group breakdown of the population of Great Britain, highlighting the four mixed categories, and their population proportions. It additionally illustrates the proportion of each group that is UK born, demonstrating the fact that the majority of those of mixed ethnicity living in Great Britain are UK born, as we might expect. Nevertheless, around 30 per cent of both the White and Black African and Other Mixed groups are not UK born. They are not the result of mixing in the UK, therefore, but

Table 8.1 The distribution of ethnic groups in Great Britain, and proportion UK born

Ethnic group	*% of overall population*	*% of group UK born*
White British	84.1	97.6
Other White	5.2	42.4
White and Black Caribbean	**0.4**	**95.5**
White and Black African	**0.2**	**70.9**
White and Asian	**0.3**	**85.2**
Other mixed	**0.2**	**69.8**
Indian	2.2	42.5
Pakistani	1.7	56.5
Bangladeshi	0.7	50.4
Other Asian	0.8	24.4
Black Caribbean	1.1	61.4
Black African	1.4	33.9
Black Other	0.1	64.3
Chinese	0.4	25.2
Other	1.4	22.1
Total (N)	100 (688,028)	89.1

Source: Quarterly Labour Force Survey, pooled quarters Q4 2003–Q3 2010.
Note: This and all subsequent tables and analyses are weighted to reflect population proportions and adjust for non-response using the appropriate person weights within the data.

reflect the complex heritages that many who come to the UK already bring with them. This means that Great Britain's mixed population cannot simply be interpreted in terms of openness to interethnic partnership of its populations both minority and majority. Indeed, some growth of the UK mixed population will be consequent on immigration, and how those immigrants choose to define themselves in the face of an increasing range of potential categories.

The predominantly UK-born profile of the mixed groups is reflected in an overwhelmingly youthful population. Given patterns of migration to the UK, the demographic profile of those children born to minorities within the UK is strongly concentrated in the younger age groups. This is shown in Table 8.2 where we can see mixed groups, the majority population and other minority groups banded by age, with over half of those of mixed ethnicity being aged under 16. This compares with only 19 per cent of the population as a whole. Even compared with other minority groups, the profile of mixed groups is young. The youthful age profile has meant that much of our understanding of 'mixedness', how it is claimed and attributed and what it means to individuals and families, necessarily derives from studies with children and young people or with the parents of mixed-ethnicity children (e.g. Aspinall 2010; Song 2010; Phoenix and Tizard 1995; Edwards and Caballero 2008; Edwards *et al.* 2010). The demography of the mixed groups also shapes their distributions in education, employment and stage of career. The latter part of the chapter will explore the extent to which the employment experience of those of mixed ethnicity is commensurate with those from the majority and other minority groups of similar age.

Educational qualifications

First, however, we examine the levels of educational qualifications across the mixed groups by age band to explore the extent to which the mixed population is achieving credentials in line with the overall population profile (Table 8.3). We also compare them with other minorities, since minority groups show

Table 8.2 Age profile of mixed groups compared with White majority and other minority groups, 2003–2010 (column %)

	Mixed groups	*White majority*	*Other minority ethnic groups*	*Other minorities excluding White*	*All*
Under 16	51.5	17.9	21.0	25.5	18.8
16 to 24	18.3	11.5	14.1	15.2	12.0
25 to 34	11.3	11.6	20.9	20.0	13.0
35 to 59	16.2	34.7	31.8	31.1	34.0
60+	2.7	24.3	12.2	8.2	22.3
Total	100	100	100	100	100

Source: Quarterly Labour Force Survey, pooled quarters Q4 2003–Q3 2010.

Table 8.3 Distribution of qualifications across mixed, majority and other minority populations by age band (column %)

	16–24			*25–34*			*35–59*		
	Mixed	*Majority*	*Other minorities*	*Mixed*	*Majority*	*Other minorities*	*Mixed*	*Majority*	*Other minorities*
Level 4+	11	13	15	42	36	37	38	29	31
Level 3	25	25	21	14	17	7	11	12	7
Level 2	28	30	20	13	20	8	15	21	11
Less than level 2	15	17	12	9	14	6	13	15	8
Other qualifications	6	3	17	11	4	29	10	7	23
No qualifications	16	13	15	11	9	13	14	17	21
Total (N)	100 (1048)	100 (54,727)	100 (10,992)	100 (636)	100 (58,460)	100 (16,645)	100 (1055)	100 (194,928)	100 (28,842)

Table 8.4 Percentage with level 4+ or no qualifications for selected mixed and other ethnic groups by age band

		White and Black Caribbean	*Black Caribbean*	*White and Asian*	*Indian*	*White majority*
25–34	Level 4+ %	29	29	51	51	36
	None %	17	12	11	8	9
35–59	Level 4+ %	29	27	44	31	29
	None %	16	15	10	23	17

distinctive patterns of educational achievement – increasingly they have greater levels of higher (graduate level) qualifications, though at the same time there are still greater rates of no qualifications. The patterns are highly distinctive by group, both among the cohorts currently passing through school (Wilson *et al.* 2005; Hills *et al.* 2010) and within the adult population (Platt 2011: Chapter 6). Table 8.4, therefore, additionally compares qualifications for selected non-mixed ethnic groups and for the White and Black Caribbean, and White and Asian mixed groups.

Table 8.3 shows that the distribution of qualifications among the mixed groups as a whole is not so dissimilar to that of the White majority population, although within the older working age group, rates of higher qualifications appear somewhat higher. Turning to Table 8.4, however, we see the dissimilarity within the mixed groups. Due to small sample sizes, this table concentrates simply on the proportions with higher (level 4 or more) and with no qualifications. It reveals that among the 25–34 age group, White and Black Caribbeans and White and Asians have directly comparable rates of qualifications to Black Caribbeans and to Indians respectively, with the rates for the White majority falling somewhere in the middle. The implication of the very high rates of higher qualifications among both the White and Asian and the Indian groups is that whatever educational resources or family backgrounds favour the educational success of Indian young people also benefit those of White and Asian mixed ethnicity: academically, this group is not penalised through having White as well as Indian parentage.

This is not to suggest that the extensively explored differences in educational achievement across the 'non-mixed' ethnic groups are well understood; nor that we are necessarily seeing a form of transmission of values that distinguishes Indian heritage from Black Caribbean heritage children. Rather, as Tikly *et al.* (2004) have shown, the intersection of ethnicity, class and location play out in complex ways for those of mixed ethnicity, with consequences for attainment. Nevertheless, there is a degree to which factors supporting or undermining achievement of particular groups, including teacher expectations, discrimination and access to economic and social resources, which impact differentially on the experience of the non-mixed groups (Platt 2011), may link the experience of mixed and non-mixed groups with shared heritage;

even if there are also specific factors that impinge upon the experience of mixed ethnicity children, including, for example, the invisibility of mixed groups in teaching and discussion (Tikly *et al.* 2004).

Among the 25–59 age group, the White and Asian rates of higher qualifications are greater than for any other group and the rates of having no qualifications are lower. This divergence from the experience of the previous comparator, the Indian group, might be explained by the fact that the Indian population will include many who are not UK born and among the non-UK-born levels of higher qualifications, particularly for women, do not match the rates among the UK born (Platt 2011: Chapter 6).

Those of mixed ethnicity can thus be seen not only to be an internally differentiated 'group', to the extent that it is meaningful to consider it a group at all, but it would appear to be differentiated in ways that map onto the educational advantage and disadvantage of the minority element of their heritage. Thus those of mixed ethnicity do not demonstrate assimilation to majority patterns, or, as some arguments would suggest, mark a part-way position between minority and majority experiences – where they might be expected to be less affected by sources of both educational advantage and disadvantage that are a feature of the corresponding non-mixed minority groups.

These variations in educational achievement should lead us to expect variation in employment outcomes for mixed groups compared with both the majority and each other. But before considering the relationship between age, education and employment, we first give some further attention to demographic profile in terms of partnership status of the mixed groups.

Marriage and cohabitation

Although partnership status itself is not an outcome that is typically of policy interest or considered germane to discussions of group welfare or the integration or exclusion of minority ethnic groups, it is clear that patterns of partnership formation and dissolution are both shaped by economic context and have economic consequences (Jenkins 2011). There would also appear to be a cultural element to particular patterns of partnership formation, such as relatively early marriage (Dale *et al.* 2006), while lone parenthood among Caribbean mothers has been the source of sustained attention (Reynolds 2005). Rates of both singledom and of lone parenthood as well as marriage have been shown to demonstrate distinctive patterns across minority ethnic groups (Nandi and Platt 2010). For those of mixed heritage, there is a priori no reason to expect that patterns of family formation would differ significantly from those prevailing across the population. Opportunity structures should not impose the same constraints as those faced by other minorities, since exposure to different groups is built into their upbringing; and given that they are already the product of partnerships which have breached ethnic divides, cultural norms or expectations around marriage coming from either side of their heritage might also be expected to be weaker. Boundaries could be expected to be more blurred and thus partnership opportunities enhanced. Qian and Lichter (2007) provided some evidence for such blurring of boundaries in the US context. However, to the extent that minoritised status restricts options and social closure is experienced by these mixed groups, they might still face differential opportunities. Preferences may also be shaped by their mixed heritage and create different expectations about appropriate or desirable partner characteristics.

As Table 8.5 shows, there are significantly lower rates of marriage/partnership among those of mixed ethnicity at all ages compared with both the majority population and other minorities. Berthoud (2005) earlier proposed that the rates of lone parenthood among Caribbean parents represented the 'modern' end of a spectrum from traditional to modern, with South Asian families being more 'traditional'. On the one hand, it might be argued that those of mixed heritage are yet more 'modern' and are at the forefront of a social order that is leaving 'traditional' patterns behind, in terms of normative expectations about cohabitation and marriage. On the other hand, marriage and partnership are widely considered to have a number of positive features, whether in relation to bringing up children or providing sharing of risks and greater economic security. Without a more in-depth investigation into partnership expectations and preferences it would be premature either to celebrate these partnership patterns as marking a revolution in family practice or to regret them as evidence of closed and heavily ethnically divided society. They invite further interrogation to better understand what inferences to draw.

Table 8.6 looks at marriage rates of White and Black Caribbeans and White and Asians compared with Black Caribbeans and Indians respectively, as well as with the White majority. Concentrating just on the age ranges 25–34 and 35–59, it seems to show that relatively low rates of marriage and cohabitation are fairly common across the mixed groups. At the same time, for the White and Black Caribbean group they are higher than for the Black Caribbean group, and for the White and Asian group they are substantially

Table 8.5 Percentage married or cohabiting among mixed, majority and other minority groups by sex and age band

		Mixed groups	*Majority*	*Other minorities*	*Other minorities excluding White*
Men	16–24	8	12	11	8
	25–34	50	61	59	58
	35–59	66	78	79	82
Women	16–24	13	19	23	19
	25–34	46	64	67	65
	35–59	48	73	69	67
All	16–24	10	15	17	13
	25–34	47	63	63	62
	35–59	57	75	74	74

Table 8.6 Percentage married or cohabiting by selected ethnic groups and age group

	White and Black Caribbean	*Black Caribbean*	*White and Asian*	*Indian*	*White British majority*
Age 25–34	39	35	45	66	63
Age 35–59	54	47	66	85	75

lower than for the Indian group. However, while they appear to be showing convergence with each other, they do not approach the rates of marriage and cohabitation among the White majority.

Economic activity

The next part of this chapter moves on to consider the economic status of the adult mixed population of the UK, and employment rates in particular. Table 8.7 illustrates the distribution of the mixed groups according to their main economic activity. Only around a quarter are in employment, but given that half are under 16, this is scarcely surprising. Nevertheless, if we explore economic activity at the different age bands, we see, from Table 8.8, that at each age band, those of mixed ethnicity have lower employment rates than the majority population and correspondingly higher rates of unemployment and studentship.

To explore these patterns a little further in comparative perspective, Table 8.9, in line with the previous analysis, shows the employment rates for White and Black Caribbean compared with Caribbean and White and Asian compared with Indian, as well as to the majority. If mixedness were truly

Table 8.7 Economic activity of mixed groups compared with majority and other minority groups (column %)

	Mixed groups	*Majority*	*Other minorities*	*Other minorities excluding White*	*Total*
Employed	26.1	41.0	38.6	34.8	40.5
Self-employed	2.9	6.3	6.4	5.4	6.3
Government training scheme	0.2	0.2	0.2	0.2	0.2
ILO unemployed	3.8	2.6	4.2	4.8	2.9
Inactive	6.5	9.4	13.4	14.8	9.9
Student	7.0	3.1	6.9	8.4	3.7
Retired	2.0	19.5	9.3	6.2	17.8
Under 16	51.5	17.9	21.0	25.5	18.8
All	100	100	100	100	100

Table 8.8 Main economic activity by age band, mixed groups compared with majority (column %)

	Age 16–24		*Age 25–34*		*Age 35–59*	
	Mixed groups	*Majority*	*Mixed groups*	*Majority*	*Mixed groups*	*Majority*
Employed (inc. self-employed)	45.6	57.1	72.6	81.2	73.7	79.7
Unemployed	12.6	10.0	6.8	4.4	5.5	2.9
Inactive	8.0	8.7	15.4	13.0	19.1	17.1
Student	33.7	24.3	5.2	1.3	1.7	0.3

reflective of openness of society and of assimilative processes at work on all levels, then we might expect the mixed groups' experiences to be closer to that of the majority than to that of those who express a single minority affiliation. The numbers become quite small for such comparisons, even with the seven years of data pooled for this analysis, which means that it only makes sense to focus on employment rates, and on studentship rates for the 16–24-year-old group when looking at discrete mixed groups. As Table 8.9 shows, while the mixed groups overall seem to tread a midway path, there seems to be somewhat greater parallels between their experience and that of the corresponding non-mixed minority than with the majority. These lower employment rates of the mixed groups occur despite the relatively positive qualifications profile across the mixed groups that we saw earlier.

The indication of lower employment rates than might be expected among the mixed groups was supported by a multivariate regression controlling for age (not illustrated). Both when qualifications were and were not included in the regression, all the mixed groups (along with the other minority groups) were less likely to be employed than the majority, and this was true for both men and women. Perhaps unsurprisingly, but nevertheless revealingly, parity of economic outcome with the majority seems to elude those of mixed ethnicity as it eludes those of other minority ethnicities. While there is no evidence of particular exclusion for mixed groups, in terms of the employment measure considered here, nevertheless, as for other minorities, educational qualifications are insufficient to gain equal employment opportunities. The routes by

Table 8.9 Percentage employed by selected ethnic group and age band

		White and Black Caribbean	*Black Caribbean*	*White and Asian*	*Indian*	*White majority*
16–24	Employed % (N)	47 (206)	36 (228)	43 (112)	39 (629)	57 (31,860)
	Student % (N)	27 (134)	35 (247)	40 (113)	44 (771)	24 (15,066)
25–34	Employed % (N)	66 (143)	65 (467)	78 (134)	79 (2060)	81 (49,839)
35–59	Employed % (N)	75 (220)	76 (1840)	75 (213)	75 (3544)	80 (163,342)

which these constraints operate are doubtless complex and reflect the structurally stratified social context where access to resources is unequally distributed and inequalities are perpetuated. Given the extensive analysis of employment outcomes across minorities, both UK born and non-UK born (Platt 2007), it would be of benefit to explore further how and why the disadvantaged outcomes of mixed groups arise and what explanatory frameworks might do justice to them. A key candidate must remain racial discrimination. There is substantial evidence that discrimination continues to play a key role in employment experiences of minority groups in the UK (Heath and Cheung 2006; Wood *et al.* 2009), even while there are many other factors that combine to shape options and opportunities (which may additionally include perceived discrimination or past experiences). This is especially the case since many of the arguments applied to other minority groups excepting race-based discrimination, such as language skills, limited networks, particular concentration in deprived locations and so on, are unlikely to apply so readily to the mixed ethnic groups.

Conclusion

This chapter has provided a brief overview of the distribution and some key characteristics of the mixed ethnicity population of Great Britain. The growth and recognition of mixed ethnicity within Great Britain has been regarded as marking the openness of UK society and of both signalling and supporting the breakdown of ethnic stratification within the country. At the same time, those of mixed ethnicity are sometimes highlighted as liminal, located outside both the mainstream and minority ethnic communities, and consequently suffering both psychological and socio-economic disadvantage. This chapter indicates that neither account is necessarily complete. First of all, the four mixed categories between them account for only 1 per cent of the population; and half of them are under 16. While the ethnic profile of young people is markedly different from that of the adult population, the contribution of those of mixed ethnicity to the UK's ethnic and cultural diversity, even if increasing, is still of such a scale that it cannot make a substantial impact on the overall population (cf. Qian and Lichter 2007 in relation to the US). Most White majority people still marry and mix with other White majority people. It will also be some time before the current mixed ethnicity children grow up and we can ascertain how this generation is faring in UK society.

Nevertheless, those affiliating with the mixed ethnic groups do not appear to be relegated to the margins of society. While there is diversity across the groups, rates of higher qualifications speak of the ability to capitalise on sources of educational advantage and to levels of achievement that overall are not far off those of the majority. On the other hand patterns of economic activity indicate higher unemployment and an employment 'penalty' for those of minority ethnicity, though some of this is down to greater retention in education than is the case for the majority. The increased levels of studentship may bring longer-term gains for the groups even if they lower employment rates in the recent period. The distributions of employment suggest that minority status accompanies those of mixed ethnicity. Whatever the constraints, employment patterns (as also for education patterns) are closer to those of the specific minority ethnicities which form part of the mixed affiliation, than they are to showing a midway point between them and the majority, or marking a separate common trajectory for those of mixed ethnicity.

In relation to arguments concerning the assimilative nature of inter-ethnic partnerships and their resulting children, the analysis in this chapter is obviously not able to draw any clear conclusions, which must await more detailed analysis. Nevertheless, the majority heritage of these mixed ethnicity individuals does not seem to imply any greater levels of economic and – to the extent that marriage is an indicator – of social integration. Indeed one of the intriguing findings of this chapter is the distinctly low marriage and cohabitation rates among those of mixed ethnicity. As the discussion above made clear, whether this is an indicator of a modern, forward-looking population, or indicative of enduring social constraints which severely limit the opportunities for partnership, requires further research.

Overall, the mixed ethnicity population of the UK represents a diversity of heritages, born of increasing partnerships between majority and minorities alongside increasing recognition in official statistics and the willingness – even enthusiasm – of individuals to assert and have acknowledged their varied antecedents. It shows that there is little evidence that those of mixed ethnicity form a group with an independently developing trajectory. At the same time, the experience of the mixed groups both collectively and individually shows distinctive traits that merit further explanation. This analysis has described some of the contours of the mixed populations and how this emergent population relates to the wider society and social structure. The experience of Britain's mixed populations seems to require a refinement of theoretical and conceptual accounts that are typically applied to minority groups to encompass the additional complexity of these patterns.

Note

1 In this analysis I concentrate on those in Great Britain, excluding the Northern Ireland sample, since the classification of ethnic groups differs in Northern Ireland and cannot be harmonised at a sufficiently detailed level for the purposes of this chapter with the rest of the UK. However, when determining whether someone is UK born I include birth in Northern Ireland.

References

Aspinall, P. (2000) 'The challenges of measuring the ethno-cultural diversity of Britain in the new millennium', *Policy and Politics*, 28(1): 109–18.

——(2003) 'The conceptualisation and categorisation of mixed race/ethnicity in Britain and North America: identity options and the role of the state', *International Journal of Intercultural Relations*, 27(3): 269–96.

——(2010) 'Concepts, terminology and classifications for the "mixed" ethnic or racial group in the United Kingdom', *Journal of Epidemiology and Community Health*, 64(6): 557–60.

Ballard, R. (1997) 'The construction of a conceptual vision: "ethnic groups" and the 1991 UK Census', *Ethnic and Racial Studies*, 20: 182–94.

Barn, R., Andrew, L. and Mantovani, N. (2005) *Life After Care: The Experiences of Young People from Different Ethnic Groups*, York: Joseph Rowntree Foundation.

Barn, R. and Harman, V. (2006) 'A contested identity: an exploration of the competing social and political discourse concerning the identification and positioning of young people of inter-racial parentage', *British Journal of Social Work*, 36(8): 1309–24.

Barth, F. (1969) *Ethnic Groups and Boundaries: The Social Organisation of Culture Difference*, London: Allen & Unwin.

Berthoud, R. (1998) 'Defining ethnic groups: origin or identity?', *Patterns of Prejudice*, 32(2): 53–63.

——(2005) 'Family formation in multicultural Britain: diversity and change' in G. C. Loury, T. Modood and S. M. Teles (eds) *Ethnicity, Social Mobility and Public Policy*, Cambridge: Cambridge University Press, pp. 222–53.

Burton, J., Nandi, A. and Platt, L. (2010) 'Measuring ethnicity: challenges and opportunities for survey research', *Ethnic and Racial Studies*, 33(8): 1332–49.

Dale, A., Lindley, J. and Dex, S. (2006) 'A life-course perspective on ethnic differences in women's economic activity in Britain', *European Sociological Review*, 22(4): 459–76.

Duncan, B. and Trejo, S. (2007) 'Ethnic identification, intermarriage, and unmeasured progress by Mexican Americans' in George J. Borjas (ed.) *Mexican Immigration to the United States*, Chicago: National Bureau of Economic Research and the University of Chicago Press, pp. 229–67.

Duncan, O. D. and Lieberson, S. (1959) 'Ethnic segregation and assimilation', *American Journal of Sociology*, 64: 364–74.

Edwards, R. and Caballero, C. (2008) 'What's in a name? An exploration of the significance of personal naming of "mixed" children for parents from different racial, ethnic and faith backgrounds', *The Sociological Review*, 56(1): 39–60.

Edwards, R., Caballero, C. and Puthussery, S. (2010) 'Parenting children from "mixed" racial, ethnic and faith backgrounds: typifications of difference and belonging', *Ethnic and Racial Studies*, 33(6): 949–67.

Finnäs, F. and O'Leary, R. (2003) 'Choosing for the children: the affiliation of the children of minority–majority group intermarriages', *European Sociological Review*, 19(5): 483–99.

Fryer, R. G. (2007) 'Guess who's been coming to dinner? Trends in interracial marriage over the 20th century', *Journal of Economic Perspectives*, 21(2): 71–90.

Furtado, D. (2006) 'Human capital and interethnic marriage decisions', IZA Discussion Paper 1989: Bonn: IZA.

Gordon, M. M. (1964) *Assimilation in American Life*, Oxford: Oxford University Press.

Harris, D. and Sim, J. J. (2002) 'Who is multi-racial? Assessing the complexity of lived race', *American Sociological Review*, 67(4): 614–27.

Heath, A. and Cheung, S.Y. (2006) 'Ethnic penalties in the labour market: employers and discrimination', Department for Work and Pensions Research Report No 34. Leeds: Corporate Document Services.

Hills, J., Brewer, M., Jenkins, S., Lister, R., Lupton, R., Machin, S., Mills, C., Modood, T., Rees, T. and Riddell, S. (2010) *An Anatomy of Economic Inequality in the UK: Report of the National Equality Panel*, London: Government Equalities Office / Centre for Analysis of Social Exclusion.

Hwang, S.-S., Saenz, R. and Aguirre, B. E. (1997) 'Structural and assimilationist explanations of Asian American intermarriage', *Journal of Marriage and the Family*, 59(3): 758–72.

Jenkins, S. (2011) *Changing Fortunes: Income Mobility and Poverty Dynamics in Britain*, Oxford: Oxford University Press.

Joppke, C. (1999) *Immigration and the Nation-State: The United States, Germany, and Great Britain*, Oxford: Oxford University Press.

Kalmijn, M. and van Tubergen, F. (2006) 'Ethnic intermarriage in the Netherlands: confirmations and refutations of accepted insights', *European Journal of Population*, 22: 371–97.

Kantarevic, J. (2004) 'Interethnic marriages and economic assimilation of immigrants', IZA Discussion Paper No. 1142. Bonn: IZA.

Meng, X. and Gregory, R. G. (2005) 'Intermarriage and the economic assimilation of immigrants', *Journal of Labor Economics*, 23(1): 135–75.

Model, S. and Fisher, G. (2002) 'Unions between blacks and whites: England and the US compared', *Ethnic and Racial Studies*, 25(5): 728–54.

Muttarak, R. and Heath, A. (2010) 'Who intermarries in Britain: explaining ethnic diversity in intermarriage pattern', *British Journal of Sociology*, 61(2): 275–305.

Nandi, A. and Platt, L. (2010) *Ethnic Minority Women's Poverty and Economic Well-Being*, London: Government Equalities Office.

Phillips, T. (2009) 'Stephen Lawrence speech: institutions must catch up with public on race issues', Speech by Trevor Phillips, Chair of the Commission to mark the tenth anniversary of the Stephen Lawrence Inquiry, 19 January 2009, *Race in Britain: Ten Years since the Stephen Lawrence Inquiry*. London: Equalities and Human Rights Commission.

Phoenix, A. and Tizard, B. (1995) 'The identity of mixed parentage adolescents', *Journal of Child Psychology and Psychiatry*, 36(8): 1399–410.

Platt, L. (2007) *Ethnicity and Poverty in the UK*, Bristol: The Policy Press.

——(2009) *Ethnicity and Family – Relationships within and between Ethnic Groups: An Analysis using the Labour Force Survey*, London: Equality and Human Rights Commission.

——(2011) *Understanding Inequalities: Stratification and Difference*, Cambridge: Polity Press.

Qian, Z-C., and Lichter, D. T. (2007). 'Social boundaries and marital assimilation: evaluating trends in racial and ethnic intermarriage', *American Sociological Review*, 72: 68–94.

Rees, P., Wohland, P., Norman, P., Boden, P. and Jasinska, M. (2010) 'Ethnic population projects for the UK and local areas, 2001–2051', School of Geography Working Paper (10/02). Leeds: University of Leeds.

Rees, P., Wohland, P., Norman, P. and Boden, P. (2011) 'A local analysis of ethnic group population trends and projections for the UK', *Journal of Population Research*, 28: 149–83.

Reynolds, T. (2005) *Caribbean Mothers: Identity and Experience in the UK*, London: The Tufnell Press.

Salt, J. (1996) 'Immigration and ethnic group' in D. Coleman and J. Salt (eds) *Ethnicity in the 1991 Census: Volume One: Demographic Characteristics of the Ethnic Minority Populations*, London: HMSO, pp. 124–50.

Song, M. (2009) 'Is intermarriage a good indicator of integration?', *Journal of Ethnic and Migration Studies*, 35(2): 331–48.

——(2010) 'Does "race" matter? A study of mixed race siblings' identifications', *Sociological Review*, 58(2): 265–85.

Tikly, L., Caballero, C., Haynes, J. and Hill, J. (2004) *Understanding the Educational Needs of Mixed Heritage Pupils*, London: DfES.

van Ours, J. C. and Veenman, J. (2008) 'How interethnic marriages affect the educational attainment of children: evidence from a natural experiment', IZA Discussion Paper No. 3308. Bonn: IZA.

Weber, M. (1978) *Economy and Society*, edited by G. Roth and C. Wittich, Berkeley: University of California Press.

Wildsmith, E., Gutmann, M. P. and Gratton, B. (2003) 'Assimilation and intermarriage for US immigrant groups, 1880–1990', *History of the Family*, 8: 563–84.

Wilson, D., Burgess, S. and Briggs, A. (2005) 'The dynamics of school attainment of England's ethnic minorities', Centre for Market and Public Organisation [CMPO] Working Paper No. 05/130: University of Bristol.

Wood, M., Hales, J., Purdon, S., Sejersen, T. and Hayllar, O. (2009) *A Test for Racial Discrimination in Recruitment Practice in British Cities, Department for Work and Pensions Research Report 607*. Leeds: Corporate Document Services.

9 'Mixed-race' young people's differential responses to misrecognition in Britain

Miri Song and Peter Aspinall

Introduction

The growth of 'mixed-race'[1] people and relationships and changes in census and other official classification of ethnic and racial groups in countries such as the US, Canada, and Britain have engendered a recent spate of studies which address the issue of how multiracial people choose their racial identifications. In this chapter, we examine the question of whether mixed-race young people believe that their chosen identifications are validated by others; we then investigate how these young people respond to others' racial perceptions of them.

Various American scholars, and Mary Waters (1990) in particular, have argued that minority people who are not White possess fewer or no ethnic options compared with White Americans, who can exercise choice about whether they are ethnic, or whether they are simply Americans. This thinking can be extended to mixed people, many of whom do not appear White, and who are thus racially assigned in ways which are beyond their control (Song 2003; Spickard 1992). Their very mixedness, and the identity options available to them, present interesting and yet under-explored areas of study, especially in the British context.

Recent evidence concerning the racial identification of Black/White mixed people suggests growing latitude in how they may identify, or be identified by others (see Rockquemore and Brunsma 2002; Khanna 2004). For example, Rockquemore and Brunsma (2002) found that around three-fifths of 'biracial' respondents chose 'border' identities, in which they refused to choose one race over another; however, their border identities were not always validated by others. Although some common themes about attributions of marginality (and pressures to 'choose sides') can apply to all mixed people, the main point of comparison which has emerged in the US literature concerns the ethnic options of Black/White versus Asian/White (and to a lesser extent, Latino/White and Native American/White) people. In their analysis of a large data set of adolescents in the US, Harris and Sim (2002) ask respondents (who identify with more than one 'race') to choose a single racial category. Harris and Sim, along with Tashiro (2002) and Herman (2004), suggest that

Asian/White people in the US may identify as *either* White or Asian, and may therefore be said to possess more latitude in their identity options than Black/White people.

Why may differential ethnic options across disparate types of multiracial people matter? In the US, from where the majority of studies of mixed-race people and experiences (or what most American scholars call 'multiracial' people) still come, the greater variability in how Asian/White individuals racially identify (and are identified) reflects not only the application of the 'one drop rule' to anyone with known Black heritage, but also the fact that non-Black mixed groups have had less difficulty in crossing colour lines (Twine and Gallagher 2008; Lee and Bean 2004). In addition to the issue of individual agency, the ethnic options of disparate mixed groups matter because they tend to reflect racial fault lines (including the social distance between specific groups), the differential values and meanings associated with disparate 'races', and society's continuing preoccupation with racial difference in everyday life. In Britain, the study of mixed-race experiences and identification, while growing, is still relatively nascent. This chapter will focus specifically upon different types of mixed-race young people in Britain, especially those in the Greater London area.

The literature on *expressed* and *observed* racial identifications

Some recent work has substantially advanced our understanding of the process of the internal–external (or expressed versus observed) dialectic of identification, extending exploration of the ground where 'self-image' meets 'public image' in relation to the mixed-race population. Harris and Sim (2002) have conceptualized the multiple nature of racial identities in terms of 'internal identities' (how we think of ourselves), 'expressed identities' (what we say we are), and 'observed identities' (what others think we are based on our appearance) (see also Nagel 1994).

The way others identify us in the context of everyday life may be determined to a large degree by our physical appearance, which is the identity attribute most readily accessible to others. The extent to which the identities held by individuals are validated by others has been comprehensively investigated in the work of Brunsma and Rockquemore (2001), which reveals a strong association between socially mediated appearance and how Black/White Americans construct their identity. In her study of Asian/White adults in the US, Khanna (2004) also found that 'reflected appraisals' – individuals' perceptions of how others see them – were very influential in shaping their racial identifications.

In the case of mixed individuals, there is evidence of disjuncture between expressed (and/or internal) and observed identifications (see Campbell and Troyer 2007; Rockquemore and Laszloffy 2005). This disjuncture between how one sees oneself, in racial terms, and how others perceive one, is a form of *misrecognition*. In other words, how one sees oneself is not validated by others (Herring *et al.* 2004; Campbell and Troyer 2007; Nagel 1994). The issue of validation is, for many, fundamental, because without validation of one's own racial identity by others, one cannot easily assert and 'own' that identity (Rockquemore and Brunsma 2002). However, in addition to the possibility that misrecognition by others can be a negative experience, another possibility which has received little attention thus far is that observed identification by others may not always figure that prominently (or is of variable importance) in how individuals come to see themselves. A further possibility is that some mixed people may even enjoy others' inability to 'place' them.

This chapter thus focuses upon the ways in which disparate types of mixed young people in Britain respond to others' racial perceptions of them and examines not only the potential disjuncture between expressed and observed identities for mixed individuals, but also *the variable ways in which mixed people may feel about how they are seen by the wider public*. Previous literature on this topic (see Townsend *et al.* 2009; Cheryan and Monin 2005) has tended to assume that the disjuncture between expressed and observed identification is problematic, but our study of multiracial people in Britain suggests that this may not always be the case for all mixed groups.

The study of 'mixed-race' young people in Britain

For the first time, the growth in multiracial people was officially recognized by the inclusion of a 'Mixed' group (encompassing four mixed sub-categories) in the 2001 England and Wales Census, through which about 661,000 people were identified as mixed, or 1.27 per cent of the population of England and Wales (Bradford 2006; Aspinall 2009).[2] Demographers have identified the mixed group as one of the fastest growing of all ethnic groups, with projections indicating a 30 per cent growth during 2010–20 to achieve a population of 1.2 million (Rees 2007).

British studies of mixed people have grown significantly, focusing upon racial identification (Aspinall 2003; Tizard and Phoenix 1993; Ali 2003; Ifekwunigwe 1999; Olumide 2002), family relationships (Caballero *et al.* 2008; Twine 2004) and child welfare (Barn 1999). But up to now, no study of different types of mixed people has been conducted in Britain, and no British study has examined the dynamic of expressed and observed identification for mixed people or how they respond to their misrecognition by others.

This chapter draws on the findings of a project funded by the Economic and Social Research Council on the ethnic options of mixed-race young people in Britain, which focused upon how young people (aged 18 to 25 in higher and further education institutions in Britain) perceived and made choices about their ethnic and racial identifications. We adopted a cross-sectional study design, with the use of a semi-structured online survey, followed by in-depth interviews with a sub-set of these survey respondents. Young adults were recruited from universities and colleges of further education across England (but primarily from London, the city with the greatest number of multiracial residents). The fact that the majority of questionnaires were returned from the Greater London area may result in a skewed experience of being 'mixed race', since this area is particularly diverse and cosmopolitan.

A stratified sample (based on location and size of the mixed-race student population) was drawn from a sampling frame that integrated ethnically coded data for students in universities and colleges supplied by the Higher Education Statistics Agency and the Learning and Skills Council. Participating institutions hosted a web-link to the online survey, and these institutions sent out an email advertising our research to its student body, so those who participated in the study self-identified as mixed race. That is, we recruited individuals who recognized their multiracial ancestry (but who did not necessarily identify in any one way, e.g. as 'mixed race'). Of the 514 surveys returned to us, only 326 were within scope of our specifications (e.g. self-ascribed as mixed race, age, and post-primary school upbringing in Britain). Most of the respondents were between 18 and 25, with 258 women and 68 men. As in other such surveys of this population, many more women than men participated in the online survey, perhaps reflecting a gendered willingness to 'talk' about identifications, or even a gendered propensity to see themselves as 'mixed', as opposed to one 'race' (Lopez 2003). From these 326 surveys, a sub-sample of 65 were then purposively recruited for an in-depth interview, in part to redress the gender imbalance. The interview sample was also drawn to be representative of the *range* of mixes identified in the survey. This chapter draws upon the data from the sub-sample of 65 interviewees.

The 65 interview respondents (27 men, 38 women) comprised:

(i) Black/White: 17 (4 men, 13 women)
(ii) South Asian/White (South Asian = e.g. Indian, Pakistani): 10 (7 men, 3 women)
(iii) East or SE Asian/White (East/SE Asian = e.g. Chinese, Filipino):[3] 16 (7 men, 9 women)
(iv) Arab/White (Arab = e.g. Iranian, Egyptian): 15 (7 men, 8 women)
(v) Minority Mix (e.g. Black and Asian): 7 (2 men, 5 women)

In this chapter, we focus upon how different groups of mixed respondents felt about how they were perceived by others. Were their racial identifications validated by others, and did it matter? While the small number of respondents in each of the five groups does not allow for a systematic analysis of group differences, the in-depth interviews provide important insights into how different types of multiracial people perceive and experience their identity options.

Findings

How groups experience misrecognition by others

As discussed in a growing number of studies (see Rondilla and Spickard 2007; Herring *et al.* 2004; Brunsma and Rockquemore 2001; Khanna 2004;

Table 9.1 How groups respond to misrecognition by others

	Negative	*Positive*	*Indifferent*
Black/White	8	2	7
East or SE Asian/White	4	7	5
Arab/White	3	1	11
South Asian/White	1	3	6
Minority Mix	1	2	4
Total = 65	17	15	33

Source: ESRC-funded 'The Ethnic Options of Mixed Race People in Britain', 2006–08 (P. Aspinall and M. Song).

Herman 2004), one's physical appearance is central to how one is perceived in ethnic and racial terms. The ways in which our multiracial respondents were seen by others could vary considerably: while some were consistently pigeon-holed into a single racial category (such as 'White', 'Asian', or 'Black'), others were seen in a multitude of ways, as *physically ambiguous* individuals who were not readily assigned to existing racial categories. For this latter group, a common theme reported in studies of mixed people is that many people did not know how to 'place' them in the existing taxonomy of racial categories.

All of the interview respondents reported that they were sometimes or regularly misrecognized by others. That is, there was a mismatch between how they saw themselves and how others saw them in racial terms. Note that self-identification is not necessarily based upon a respondent's *actual* parentage; so misrecognition could occur whenever others' perceptions clashed with how one *wished to be seen*. We relied upon respondents' own reports of how others saw them. We did so by asking them (a) how others saw them in racial terms, including the ways in which they were misrecognized by others; (b) how they felt about how others perceived them. In the interviews, we asked respondents for specific examples of how they were seen by others, and how this made them feel.

While misrecognition was widely reported across all the mixed groups, their responses to this misrecognition tended to vary according to three possible responses (see Table 9.1): (a) for some, the disparity between how others saw them and how they saw themselves posed a regular source of irritation or stress in their day-to-day lives; (b) for some, others' misrecognition of them was actually experienced positively, not negatively; (c) yet others were reportedly indifferent to how others saw them, and did not pay much attention to, or take seriously, others' perceptions of them. Rather than attempting to discern whether our respondents were actually accurate about how other people racially assigned them or not (which would not be possible, retrospectively), we wanted to see *the ways in which respondents felt misrecognized by others, and how this made them feel.*

Of the 65 respondents, 17 reported that the ways in which others saw them was problematic, and chafed against their racial assignment by others. By comparison, 15 respondents were positive about how they were seen, overall (despite the fact that they were often misrecognized). What was most notable, however, was that 33 respondents claimed to be indifferent to how they were perceived by others. These respondents simply did not seem to care about how they were seen in terms of their 'race'.

Negative experiences of misrecognition

For 17 respondents (eight Black/White, one Black/Asian, three Arab/White, four East or SE Asian/White, and one South Asian/White) others' misrecognition of them was seen as problematic. How others racially assigned them jarred with how they saw themselves, and this was a recurring concern in their day-to-day lives. Significantly, eight Black/White respondents and one Black/East Asian respondent objected to the fact that they were usually seen as Black, as opposed to mixed. One of these respondents, Carrie, had a Black African mother and White English father, and saw herself as being mixed race. Yet she felt that her mixed identity was rarely validated, by either Black or White people:

> It annoys me, because I can't control it. Black people want me to say I'm Black and if I don't, I'm supposedly ashamed to be Black. Some White people will just say I'm Black, without thinking also. I hate being generalized, and it gets harder I think as you get older.

Few people validated her mixed identity, and Carrie felt highly annoyed and constrained by other peoples' insistence that she was Black. And although she did not see herself as White, she was bothered by the fact that being White was clearly off limits to her. The reported inaccessibility of either a White or a 'mixed' identity for Black/White individuals like Carrie was pronounced.

Tara, one of our 'Minority Mix' respondents, objected to others' (both White and Black peoples') perception of her as Black, and the expected script of behaviour this racial assignment entailed. Tara had a Sierra Leonian father and a Malaysian mother, and she considered herself to be 'mixed race' and 'Afro-Asian' – a hybrid identification recognizing both sides of her heritage. Because she grew up in a middle-class, predominantly White suburb of London, she reported that she was very comfortable around White people, and that she did not think about being 'different' in most contexts. Yet Tara was aware that most White people saw her as Black, and she felt constrained by other peoples' expectations that she behave in a particular way: 'My [White] friends say I'm the Whitest Black person they know.' Although she was simply being herself, her White friends at university perceived her as acting against type – since she was seen primarily as a Black person. Tara was also upset by some Black peoples' expectations that she act more 'Black'. All of these respondents objected to what they perceived as a negation of their individuality – they were simply perceived as racial types.

While in the minority among East or SE Asian/White respondents, George, who was Chinese and White English, complained of being seen 'only' as a Chinese person, because he saw himself as very British. He'd had hardly any exposure to Chinese culture and people, and had grown up in a mostly White northern city, where he had 'stuck out like a sore thumb'. Based upon his appearance (though his name was wholly Anglo), he had encountered a lot of racial taunting at school, and was highly aware of the fact that the 'public' saw him as a non-White foreigner. This treatment angered and depressed him. His experiences of racism had made him all the more determined to assert his White British side:

> You will probably not find anyone more patriotic than me or my brother. … We're super patriotic. … It's a repeated bitterness actually to be honest, because it's that thing of trying as hard as you can to be British and never having done anything else, and then realizing that that life is always going to be beyond your control.

Thus, while many East and SE Asian/White respondents like George saw themselves as British (though not necessarily 'White' in racial terms), this was not always validated by others, given his 'Chinese' physical appearance (Song and Hashem 2010). As another Chinese/White respondent, Alison, noted, 'I'm often asked where I'm from – this implicitly denies me the right to be British because of the way I look.'

Problematic experiences of being misrecognized also arose for a minority of respondents who were seen as White. In comparison to those who were only seen in relation to their non-White ancestries, four of the respondents who reported that they were consistently misrecognized complained of being seen as *White*, though they did not identify in this way. For instance, Miriam, who had a Palestinian mother and Belgian father, was blonde and blue-eyed, and this made her assertion of Arab identity very difficult, not only in relation to the public, but also with her Arab relatives:

> It's also very difficult in a family to not look the same [as others], to not be seen as an Arab fully … it does play a big role in how I identify myself and why I choose to call myself an Arab. It's more to say, well, I am here too, you know, I do count.

These respondents encountered outright incredulity (and sometimes hostility) when they claimed their minority ancestries. Because they felt a very strong attachment to their minority backgrounds, scepticism about their minority ancestry was often painful. Thus although they were not insensitive to the privileges they enjoyed as a result of a White appearance, racial misclassification as White was distressing to these respondents.

In addition to those who were racially assigned by others into a single category (White or minority), some respondents objected to the fact that others constantly saw them as *physically indeterminate*. While none of them was consistently pigeon-holed into a single racial category, and while they did not expect 'the public' to discern how they identified themselves, they commonly reported irritation about constant questioning (and scepticism) concerning their heritage: 'Where are you from?', 'What are you?' For these people, such questioning was intrusive and suggestive of unwelcome attributions of difference, based upon their ambiguous and 'foreign' appearance. Claims to being British were also sometimes challenged, and these respondents felt that they had to explain their backgrounds when they had no wish to do so.

Positive about how they were seen by others

In comparison with the 17 respondents who found other peoples' perceptions of them to be very problematic, 15 of the 65 interviewees articulated primarily positive experiences about how they were seen (albeit often misrecognized) by others. Seven of these 15 were East or SE Asian/White, three South Asian/White, one Arab/White, two 'Minority Mix', and two Black/White. These respondents, most of whom were seen as physically indeterminate, reported that they enjoyed the fact that people were unable to discern their ethnic and racial heritage.

Many of these respondents, and in particular female respondents, said that they enjoyed the attention they received from others because of their physical ambiguity – they were considered 'exotic'. The guessing game involved in people's reactions to them was often a good 'conversation starter'. As one male respondent put it, 'The girls love it!'. Hari (Indian and White English) said that his physical appearance aroused curiosity: 'I quite like it because … it's like it makes me a bit more, I suppose, mysterious. It's sort of quite glamorous … Yeah, from my point of view it's quite nice, that sort of uniqueness.' Although some male respondents, such as Hari, reported that they liked being seen as exotic, the awareness that being mixed, and thus physically alluring, appeared to be gendered.

Like Hari, looking physically ambiguous also made Jenny (Chinese and White English), feel special and attractive: 'To be honest, my sister and I look quite similar and were quite cute when we were kids, and it was often, "Aren't you pretty", it was never negative.' Crucially, the curiosity they encountered was experienced positively, in contrast to the respondents (who were seen as physically indeterminate) who reported negative attributions of being foreign or odd looking. Some of the respondents who felt positive about how they were seen by others articulated thoughts which were reminiscent of those expressed in Waters' (1990) study of White Americans, in which many White Americans tried to highlight an ethnic ancestry (e.g. Irish, Italian, Polish) in order to feel more distinctive, and not 'just' American.

In none of these cases did these respondents feel racialized as outsiders in Britain; in other words, their perceived difference by others was not one which elicited xenophobic notions of not belonging in the nation. For instance, Brad (Sri Lankan and White English) talked of how he felt very much at home in Britain, and accepted as British, too. Yet he noted that his 'ambiguous' (his words) physical appearance provided him with a variety of ethnic options:

> If I'm outside of the UK then people say where are you from? And I'll be English or from the UK or British. … Because I realize that I'm all of those things. I realize that at college I have quite a lot friends from, most of my male friends are from India or other parts of Asia … but then I am also more White with other people, too. So I dunno, it's quite flexible.

While Brad felt completely at home in Britain (and this sense of belonging was not challenged), he also enjoyed the fact that he was able to claim an affinity to 'India or other parts of Asia' at university.

Although most of these respondents were unable to control how others saw them, and could not effectively invoke specific identifications at will, they enjoyed the fact that they were not easily categorized – in stark contrast with the Black/White respondents who identified as mixed, but felt pigeon-holed into the Black category. For these respondents, misrecognition by others could be a source of fun or amusement because (a) their sense of belonging in Britain was primary (and secure); these individuals were not heavily invested in a specific ethnic or racial identity, whether it be Chinese, Barbadian, Black, or Asian, to name a few; (b) how others racially assigned them was not considered to be stigmatizing – rather, the fact that others found it difficult to 'place them' made them feel special and distinctive.

Indifferent to how they were seen by others

In comparison to respondents who reported either negative or positive experiences in terms of how others perceived them, 33 of the 65 interview respondents (comprising seven of 17 Black/White, 11 of 15 Arab/White, six of 10 South Asian/White, five of 16 East or SE Asian/White, and four of seven 'minority mix') claimed to be indifferent to how they were seen by other people. A large number of these respondents talked about the fact that although they were often misrecognized, they were not terribly concerned about how others saw them in racial terms.

This lack of concern derived from the fact that their 'race' was not particularly central to their sense of self and/or the fact that their race was less salient than their overriding sense of Britishness, or their religion, studies, or regional identification (e.g. as a Londoner). This derogation of racial difference was typically mentioned in terms of everyday life in large urban centres like London. As one South Asian/White respondent, Ben, put it, 'You don't really expect people to be White in London!' Or as Kareem (Pakistani and Arab) observed, 'I am what I am … I'm just technically another person just walking.' Nor did they think that their peers paid much attention to their exact parental heritage, given their common upbringing as British.

Beth (Black African and English) refused to racially identify, claiming that she transcended categorization. She also reported that she was seen in many different ways, ranging from 'mixed race', to Mediterranean and Middle Eastern, but that she was not worried about how other people saw her:

> I personally forget most of the time that I have an ethnicity, but I am lucky to have been successful academically and study in a world where I don't feel that such things are important. … as I say, it's not an issue that even occurs to me unless someone raises it.

As a child, she had grown up in a northern town, and had lived in a predominantly White neighbourhood, in which she had felt consciously different, being part-Black. But in London, where she had lived for the last 10 years, she reported that she felt very ordinary. Unlike Beth (who transcended racial identification), there were some Black/White respondents who identified as mixed or Black, but who also claimed that they did not particularly care how others saw them.

Peter (Vietnamese and White English) identified as a 'mixed' person. He said that he had been seen as ambiguous – sometimes South American, 'Oriental', or Mexican, but how others saw him did not matter very much to him. Although he had felt different and 'vulnerable' (in terms of being racially targeted) in primary school, he did not pay much attention to how others now saw him, even though he could encounter occasional racial prejudice: 'When I think of me, I don't think. … The first thing is not race. It's not an issue.' While he would readily note his parental heritage on official forms, his racial and ethnic heritage did not figure centrally to how he saw himself.

Of course, claimed indifference to how they were seen in racial terms should not necessarily be taken at face value. In comparison to those Black/White respondents who were consistently seen as 'Black' (and who experienced this racial assignment in a negative way), it is relatively easy for respondents who are not consistently pigeon-holed (or who may 'pass') to claim that race is not an issue (Waters 1990; Song 2003). Nevertheless, there were a significant number of respondents across all the multiracial groups (most of whom did not appear White), including some who were consistently seen as Black (but who saw themselves as being 'mixed'), who reported that they were indifferent to how they were seen by others.

Such a claimed indifference to how others racially assigned them did not necessarily mean that these respondents had not experienced forms of racism, but they were able to contain and minimize the significance of such negative experiences. Even so, most of these respondents recognized the contextually specific ways in which being 'different' could matter, especially in settings outside multiethnic London, where one could, as one respondent put it, be outside one's 'comfort zone'.

Discussion and conclusion

A growing body of research in the US and Britain has investigated the racial identifications of multiracial people. While large-scale surveys in the US have provided valuable overviews of how different types of 'mixed' people racially identify themselves, previous studies of mixed-race people in Britain have not investigated the variation of experiences across disparate multiracial groups. Through the use of in-depth interviews with 65 British respondents, we explored how mixed-race young people responded to their racial assignment by others. Below are our four main findings:

Indifference to misrecognition

This research extends existing studies by examining not only the potential disjuncture between expressed and observed identities for mixed individuals, but also *the variable ways in which mixed people may feel about how they are seen by the wider public*. Misrecognition was not problematic for all our respondents, with some people experiencing this misrecognition very negatively, others positively, and yet others, with indifference. Crucially, such variation in responses to misrecognition was found both across and within all the mixed groups.

How should we interpret this reported indifference to misrecognition? In addition to the fact that they did not *expect* the wider public to validate their expressed identifications, these respondents tended to note (a) the fact that they were British, regardless of 'colour', and (b) the relative unimportance of race in cosmopolitan, metropolitan settings such as London, where degrees of conviviality and mixing were high, and where being of any hue or mixture was regarded as unremarkable – at least in many situations. Importantly, claims to indifference were not devoid of a recognition of continuing forms of racial prejudice and disadvantage, especially in certain institutional contexts; so these claims should not be interpreted as naïve denials of the existence of 'colour-blind' racism. It may be that, in Britain, the constitution of racial identities is interwoven with other dimensions of identification and belonging that are important, such as national identity, and other modes of belonging, especially in cosmopolitan urban centres where ethnic and racial diversity is relatively commonplace.

Group differences

Despite the fact that a substantial proportion of respondents across all the groups reported indifference to others' misrecognition of them, we found differences between groups in terms of how they responded to other peoples' misrecognition of them. In comparison with the other 'mixed' groups, a higher proportion of part-Black respondents reported negative experiences and feelings about being misrecognized than any other group (the second highest was East and SE Asian/White respondents). Although the majority of the Black/White respondents saw themselves as 'mixed race', many of them were pigeon-holed as Black (as found in the US). Certainly no such rule applied to the other types of mixes in our study, so that they were less likely to be consistently pigeon-holed into a single category, such as 'Black'.

By comparison, non-Black mixed respondents were often seen to be physically indeterminate, and racially assigned in a wide variety of ways. This was experienced negatively by some, while their physical ambiguity (to others) was associated with indifference or with positive social values and encounters. A key distinction between respondents who experienced their misrecognition positively, as opposed to negatively, is that the former (a) did not expect others to validate their expressed identifications; and (b) did not perceive their racial assignment by others to entail racial prejudice or negative social value.

Nationality and Britishness

In addition to the categories of multiracial identification found by Rockquemore and Brunsma (2002), based upon Black/White individuals in the US, we would add a national mode of identification (e.g. British), in which one's sense of national belonging can take precedence over ethnic or racial identifications in many social situations – though national and racial (and ethnic) identifications are not mutually exclusive. Many of our respondents, especially non-Black mixed respondents, described themselves in terms of nationality and cultural belonging in Britain, and saw their nationality as being more salient than their racial or ethnic identities. The public did not readily recognize non-Black mixed people in racial terms, so there was no consistent way in which they were racially assigned (though this did not mean they were not subject to negative forms of racialization); furthermore, most of these young people did not feel that they could claim an ethnically authentic affiliation with some distant ancestral culture in Hong Kong or Pakistan.

While their sense of belonging in Britain seemed no less strong for part-Black respondents, their consistent and persistent racial assignment as Black by the wider public meant that they were regularly reminded of their 'race' (though some Black/White respondents managed to deflect or disregard this). Nevertheless, it is important not to overstate group differences in expressed identification between part-Black (e.g. as 'mixed race') and non-Black groups (e.g. as 'British/White British') – because despite differences in expressed identifications and experiences of feeling misrecognized, a shared sense of being British was a strong undercurrent across all the mixed groups, and served to dilute the force of differently expressed racial identifications. In this respect, given the more inclusive umbrella of national belonging we found in this study, it is a salutary reminder of avoiding a transplantation of US models or findings onto the British context – though such national inclusiveness is less likely in more predominantly White suburban and rural settings.

Differential ethnic options

In their study of how various multiracial adolescents in the US racially identify, various analysts found that, in comparison with Black/White young people, their Asian/White respondents effectively possessed a wider range of identity options. Based on our findings, the identity options of Black/White respondents in Britain (as measured by negative experiences of being misrecognized) also appear to be more constrained than those for other mixed groups. However, we need to qualify a stark comparison between part-Black versus non-Black mixed people in Britain. The fact that one is not consistently pigeon-holed into a category (as in the case of East or SE Asian/White individuals) did not automatically translate into an ability to assert a racial identification which was *validated* by others. Therefore, the apparent range of ethnic options held by non-Black mixed individuals may obscure the fact that their Britishness can be challenged, and that they can be attributed racially stigmatizing qualities.

While respondents who were seen as physically ambiguous, and thus difficult to racially assign, were not pigeon-holed into one category, some of these respondents could feel upset and 'othered' by people's unwanted attribution of foreignness and 'difference'. Variation in physical appearance within groups (e.g. East or SE Asian/White) could be considerable. Some in the South Asian/White and East or SE Asian/White categories can look mostly White, while others look much more Asian by prevailing social norms. The fact that there are no widespread social conventions in Britain about how to classify these part-Asian (or part-Arab) groups does not necessarily mean that such individuals are able to assert their desired identifications.

Thus, how respondents felt about others' misrecognition of them depended upon *the nature and implications of the misrecognition (e.g. negative meanings and stereotypes associated with specific groups)*, which tended to vary according to group membership, and was not just due to differences in individual predisposition (though of course, this, along with other factors, clearly influenced how these young people reacted to others' perceptions of them). Thus, certain forms of misrecognition were more negatively experienced and charged than others, especially for some Black/White individuals; this suggests that while there is growing intermarriage and 'conviviality' among White and Black Britons, this racial boundary is still keenly observed in particular ways, suggesting that, as in the US, there is less of a marked social distance recognized between White and other types of (non-Black) minority Britons. At the same time, we must qualify our understanding of other (e.g. part-Asian) mixed people's (limited) ethnic options.

While we did not discuss in detail other influences on identity choices, such as social class and contextual factors like the ethnic composition of respondents' neighbourhoods and the schools they attended, future studies of multiracial people need to probe the potentially significant role of social class and these other factors in shaping how multiracial individuals perceive and negotiate their identity options (Caballero *et al.* 2008). Coming from a relatively privileged background by virtue of being in higher or further education, many of our respondents may have been insulated from a sense that they lacked control over how other people perceived them.

The increasing rates of intermarriage for Black Britons (and also for Chinese and Indian Britons) with Whites suggests that being 'mixed' may become increasingly unremarkable (Song 2009). As articulated by many of the respondents in this study, it is possible that, at least in particular regions and contexts, which are multiethnic and cosmopolitan, being 'mixed' may be increasingly ordinary – though this will vary across different localities and regions. Furthermore, the meanings attached to being 'mixed', and to racial identification more generally, are fluid and changeable over time, and according to specific contexts. This increasing diversity in the demographic composition of the population, however, cannot be assumed to presage a straightforward erosion of racial awareness or racial prejudice toward mixed people.

Notes

1 While it is acknowledged that no one term is accepted by all mixed-race persons, the term 'mixed race' is used in this chapter as it was the most common term of choice identified by respondents in this study.

2 In the England and Wales 2001 Census the term 'Mixed' is the overarching term used for the four ethnic background mixed categories: 'White and Black Caribbean', 'White and Black African', 'White and Asian', and a free text 'Any other mixed background'. At the time of writing, the 2011 Census has just been disseminated, in which the 'Mixed' category of 2001 has been changed to 'Mixed/ multiple ethnic groups', with the same four subgroups listed underneath.

3 The East or SE Asian group encompasses 'Chinese and White' and mixes of other East or SE Asian origins and White, such as 'Japanese and White', 'Malaysian and White' and so on.

References

Ali, S. 2003. *Mixed-Race, Post-Race: Gender, New Ethnicities and Cultural Practices*, Oxford: Berg.

Aspinall, P. 2003. 'The conceptualisation and categorisation of mixed race/ethnicity in Britain and North America', *International Journal of Intercultural Relations* 27 (3): 269–96.

——2009. 'Does the British state's categorisation of "mixed race" meet public policy needs?', *Social Policy and Society* 9 (1):55–69.

Barn, R. 1999. 'White mothers, mixed parentage children and child welfare', *British Journal of Social Work* 29 (2): 269–84.

Bradford, B. 2006. *Who are the 'Mixed' Ethnic Group*? London: Office for National Statistics.

Brunsma, D.L. and Rockquemore, K.A. 2001. 'The new color complex: appearances and biracial identity', *Identity* 1 (3): 225–46.

Caballero, C., Edwards, R., Smith, D. 2008. 'Cultures of mixing: understanding partnerships across ethnicity', *21st Century Society* 3 (1): 49–63.
Campbell, M.E. and Troyer, L. 2007. 'The implications of racial misclassification by observers', *American Sociological Review* 72: 750–65.
Cheryan, S., and Monin, B. 2005. '"Where are you really from?": Asian Americans and identity denial', *Journal of Personality and Social Psychology* 89: 717–30.
DaCosta, K. 2007. *Making Multiracials: State, Family and Market in the Redrawing of the Color Line*, Stanford, CA: Stanford University Press.
Harris, D.R. and Sim, J.J. 2002, 'Who is multiracial? Accessing the complexity of lived race', *American Sociological Review* 67: 614–27.
Herman, M. 2004. 'Forced to choose: some determinants of racial identification in multiracial adolescents', *Child Development* 73 (3): 730–48.
Herring, C., Keith, V.M., and Horton, H.D. (eds). 2004. *Skin Deep: How Race and Complexion Matter in the 'Color-Blind' Era*, Urbana, IL: University of Illinois Press.
Ifekwunigwe, J. 1999. *Scattered Belongings*, London: Routledge.
Khanna, N. 2004. 'The role of reflected appraisals in racial identity', *Social Psychological Quarterly* 67 (2): 115–31.
Lee, J. and Bean, F. 2004. 'America's changing color lines', *Annual Review of Sociology* 30: 221–42.
Lopez, A. 2003. 'Collecting and tabulating race/ethnicity data with diverse and mixed heritage populations: a case-study with US high school students', *Ethnic and Racial Studies* 26 (5): 931–61.
Mahtani, M. and Moreno, A. 2001. 'Same difference: towards a more unified discourse in "mixed race" theory', in D. Parker and M. Song (eds) *Rethinking 'Mixed Race'*, London: Pluto Press, pp. 65–75.
Nagel, J. 1994. 'Constructing ethnicity', *Social Problems* 41 (1): 152–76.
Office for National Statistics. 2005. *Focus on Ethnicity and Identity: Inter-Ethnic Marriage*. London: Office for National Statistics. See: http://www.statistics.gov.uk/cci/nugget.asp?id=1090 Accessed 1 June 2009.
Olumide, G. 2002. *Raiding the Gene Pool*, London: Pluto Press.
Owen, C. 2007. 'Statistics: the mixed category in Census 2001', in J. Sims (ed.), *Mixed Heritage: Identity, Policy, Practice*, London: Runnymede Trust, pp. 1–5.
Rees, P. 2007. 'Ethnic population projections: review and illustration of issues'. Paper presented to Ethnic Population Projections Workshop, Cathie Marsh Centre for Census and Survey Research, May.
Rockquemore, K.A. and Brunsma, D.L. 2002. *Beyond Black: Biracial Identity in America*, Thousand Oaks, CA: Sage.
Rockquemore, K.A. and Laszloffy, T.A. 2005. *Raising Biracial Children*, Lanham, MD: AltaMira Press.
Rondilla, J. and Spickard, P. 2007. *Is Lighter Better? Skin-Tone Discrimination Among Asian Americans*, Lanham, MD: Rowman & Littlefield Publishing.
Root, M. (ed.). 1996. *The Multiracial Experience: Racial Borders as the New Frontier*, Thousand Oaks, CA: Sage.
Song, M. 2003. *Choosing Ethnic Identity*, Cambridge: Polity Press.
——2009. 'Is intermarriage a good indicator of integration?', *Journal of Ethnic and Migration Studies* 35 (2): 331–48.
Song, M. and Hashem, F. 2010 'What does "White" mean? Interpreting the choice of race by mixed race young people in Britain', *Sociological Perspectives* 53 (2): 287–92.

Spickard, P. 1992 'The illogic of racial categories', in M. Root (ed.) *Racially Mixed People in America*, Thousand Oaks, CA: Sage, pp. 12–23.

Tashiro, C. 2002. 'Considering the significance of ancestry through the prism of mixed-race identity', *Adv Nursing Science* 25 (2): 1–21.

Tizard, B. and Phoenix, A. 1993. *Black, White or Mixed Race?* London: Routledge.

Townsend, S.M., Markus, H.R. and Bergsieker, H.B. 2009. 'My choice, your categories: the verification or denial of multiracial identities', *Journal of Social Issues* 65 (1): 185–204.

Twine, F.W. 2004. 'A white side of black Britain: the concept of racial literacy', *Ethnic and Racial Studies* 27 (6): 878–907.

Twine, F.W. and Gallagher, C. 2008. *Ethnic and Racial Studies*, London: Routledge.

Waters, M.C. 1990. *Ethnic Options: Choosing Identities in America*, Berkeley, CA: University of California Press.

10 How national context shapes international comparison of 'mixed' people

The example of German, French and British large-scale survey datasets

Anne Unterreiner

Introduction

Research knowledge about 'mixed' people depends on the questions about that topic asked by researchers. But the society in which researchers are embedded influences how they conceptualize the topic, and the material that is available to them about the population they want to study.

Over time different myths are built up about how a nation came into existence and who is part of it and who is not (Anderson, 2006). Social boundaries of the particular in- and out-groups in that society – that is, the national conception of the border between 'Us' and 'Them' – thus provide the foundation for how a 'mixed' person is defined (Merton, 1964). Similarly, discussion of 'mixed' couples is based on assumptions about the existence of defined social groups and criteria for deciding who falls within and outside of them. Such criteria vary in time and space, around, variously, nationality, race, ethnicity, religion, language, culture and so on. The definition of mixedness is a social construct and its operationalisation varies from one society to another.

Mixed people are difficult to study in a comparative perspective, first because they need to be identified according to comparable criteria and second because their sample size is often small, especially in international datasets where the sample size of each country is restricted. Mixed people are often seen as part of the second or third generation of migrants. But few quantitative surveys allow for an international comparison of this second generation. The EFFNATIS survey, 'Effectiveness of National Integration Strategies towards Second-Generation Migrant Youth', conducted in 2000, counts among the few exceptions, and drew the conclusion that, '[m]arked national differences were found, but also some European convergences which are connected to all states being welfare states' (EFFNATIS, 2001, p. 7). Thus the importance of national context has been highlighted in undertaking international comparison. Moreover, because data has been collected on different ethnic group categories in different countries, comparability across countries is difficult. National contexts indeed influence the integration process of migrants and their descendents but also immigration to the country itself.

Rich contextual information is necessary to compare mixed people using large-scale datasets, especially when doing secondary analyses. Just as national context strongly influences the study of mixedness because it shapes researchers' thinking, it also determines the categorization of data in large-scale surveys. The choice of questions made by the producers of large-scale datasets is influenced by national history, national laws and national conceptions of the 'Other'. In this chapter, I take the examples of, in turn, Germany, France and Britain to explore how quantitative surveys are shaped by their specific national contexts, and draw some conclusions about the impact of this on the possibilities for cross-national comparison of populations of mixed origin. Each national case will be analysed to show, compare and contrast, the process of how social and political context over time shapes the different variables and available datasets allowing the study of mixed people.

Germany: from denial to integration

It has long been impossible to identify mixed people in large-scale datasets in Germany. This inability is first rooted in the fact that migrants were considered to be temporary workers. Second, the national myth did not fit with the reality of German state borders. As I explain below, only when Germany was reunified was the question of the integration of people of 'foreign' origin raised. Even now, the few quantitative surveys that do allow the identification of mixed people do not take ethnicity into account but at best provide the citizenship of parents, country of birth or migration status. In this context, 'mixed' is associated with and derived from parental migration path.

Historically, the use of large-scale datasets to study mixed people in Germany has been limited because the problem of how to define the German nation was not solved. Germany is a young nation-state, originating in 1871, whose territorial boundaries were subject to frequent changes with important implications. The German Empire was viewed as an incomplete nation-state because of the definition of the German nation as an ethnic and cultural community intellectually and politically (Green, 1999, p. 30). All those considered members of the German *Volk* ('folk') thus were not part of the same state. As a consequence, the Nationality Act of 1913 defined German nationality according to the *jus sanguinis* (principle of descent). Anyone who had German nationality, or was a descendant of an ethnic German, or who lived in the German Empire as it existed in 1937, was German. This ethnic conception of the German nation helps explain why the national Census treated language as the key boundary between in- and out-groups up until 1933. In the 1939 Census this boundary was extended to nationality and racial background as well as language (Labbé, 1998).This definition of German citizenry was maintained in article 116 of the West German Basic Law because, 'West Germany understood itself as a provisional state geared toward national reunification, and as homeland for the repressed and dispersed ethnic German diasporas in the Soviet empire' (Joppke, 2000, p. 152).

Any modification of German citizenship was seen as a threat to the desired unification of the two German states.

The unresolved national question meant that research on refugees, expellees and ethnic Germans that was carried out up to the late 1950s remained separate from the later body of 'guest-worker research', soon renamed 'foreigner research' (Bommes, 2010, p. 133). In the 1960s–70s, this field focused on what was viewed as the specific 'social problems' of migrants' descendents (education, health, housing and so on) (*ibid.*, p. 135). And subsequently, in the 1980s, what became called 'migration research' concerned social integration rather than ethnic minorities. Bommes highlights the fact that, because German state policy focused on foreigners rather than ethnic minorities and the recruitment of low-qualified migrants, there was no political mobilization of migrants as minorities. The 'ethnic foundation of German citizenship' and the taboo of building a politics based on the nation's conception of itself for 'historical reasons', meant that the German welfare state aimed for the social integration of foreigners rather than their political integration (*ibid.*, pp. 143–44).

At the same time as the national question was resolved through German reunification, an increase in asylum seekers and new labour migration processes, and in social tensions perceived as connected with migration, meant that migration became a major political topic in Germany. German citizenship was not the guarantor of the unification of the German nation any more, so nationality acts could be reformed 'as a tool of immigrant integration' (Joppke, 2000, p. 153). The 1990 Foreigner Law softened the 1913 Law and eased access to German nationality. But as xenophobic tensions increased and a posited 'failed integration' of young foreigners became a political, media and academic focus, a further reform of the nationality act was announced in 1998. A lively debate and political horse-trading focused on the issue of dual citizenship. This resulted in the introduction of an 'option model' in 2000, whereby, when they are aged between 18 and 23, every second-generation immigrant born in 2000 or after with two foreign parents has to choose between taking either German citizenship or that of their parents. Nationality based on place of birth, *jus soli*, was then introduced in Germany. To study mixed people in Germany, then, it is necessary to take into account the migrant trajectory of the parents rather than their current citizenship.

This new social and political context deeply influenced research on migration. Public and semi-private institutions made a stream of research funding available and the field of 'migration research' was institutionalized (Bommes, 2010, pp. 148–49). In this new research field, *Aussiedler*, 'ethnic Germans living in the former Soviet Union and Eastern and Central Europe and eligible to be accepted as citizens in Germany' (Klekowski von Koppenfels, 2009, p. 103), have been positioned as migrants in the same way as *Ausländer* (foreigners). In other words, both *Aussiedler* and *Ausländer* and their descendents are now considered as migrants, or 'people with a migration background'. As a result, the focus is not on *Ausländer* but on 'people with a migration background'. This shift led to the acknowledgement by researchers and politicians that the categories enshrined in law did not fit with social reality. There was recognition of the need for large-scale datasets with new variables, accompanied by the start of reflection on how to define people with a foreign background. Since the mid-2000s, there has been an increased political demand for statistics on the integration of migrants and their descendants as well as statistics on the effectiveness of integration policies. That is why the purpose of current research being conducted on people with a migrant background in Germany largely investigates their integration, rather than the discrimination they experience, despite the creation of institutions aiming to fight discrimination. Even though researchers tend to look beyond the administrative categories, the weight of history limits the production of large-scale datasets. Indeed, Germany's past, and especially the use to which sensitive data was put during the Third Reich, means that fear of being categorized remains high today, and that quantitative surveys where migration background is asked are still scarce (Simon, 2007). And such a limit has consequences for the identification of mixed people in large-scale datasets.

Overall citizenship is not a sufficient basis for distinguishing between people of German and of foreign background in working with large-scale survey data. When it comes to ascertaining current nationality, those with foreign parents born in Germany after 2000, *Ausländer* born in Germany, *Aussiedler* or naturalized people, cannot be distinguished from people without any migration background. This means that researchers who wish to study mixed people in Germany have to rely on information about their parents' migration biography. Nevertheless the variable collected most frequently is their current nationality (Birth Statistics, the Socio-Economic Panel SOEP,[1] *Integrationssurvey*). Looking at the specific datasets: among those constructed from public registers, the *Statistik der Geburten* (Birth Statistics) provides information about the religion and nationality of the parents of every newborn in Germany at the time of his/her birth. But the current nationality of the parents is not sufficient to distinguish between descendents of *Aussiedler*, of naturalized people and of Germans without any migration path. Information on parents' nationality, country of birth, as well as the migration status asked since 1994 are available for all respondents whose parents also took part in the SOEP survey. For other respondents, a question on parents' country of birth was added for new entrants in 2006, and parents' religion is available in this dataset. The *Integrationssurvey* 2000 does ask in which country an individual's parents were born, their current citizenship and when they arrived in Germany. That said, the construction of this survey limits its usefulness in studying mixed people as a whole population. First, it concerns people aged between 18 and 30 who are of German, Italian or Turkish origin. Second, survey participants are identified through the phonebook on the basis of the family name of the head of household, resulting in an over-representation of mixed people who have a foreign father in the Italian and

Turkish subsamples, while some mixed people having a foreign mother are located in the German one (Haug, 2004). Thus, research on mixed people in Germany is limited. In the *Mikrozensus* 2005 for example, if both generations were not considered as living in the same household, people were asked whether their parents came to Germany in 1960 or later. If so, the year of arrival in Germany and the citizenship of the parents were asked. If not, the migration path, if any, of the parents remains unknown. But because such a constraint deeply limited the study of people with a migration background, the *Mikrozensus* 2009 asked, as in the *Mikrozensus* 2005, whether their parents came to Germany in 1960 or later. If it was not the case, it was asked whether the parents were born in Germany or came prior to 1960, or whether they were not born in Germany and never came there. In addition, precise questions on parents' nationality were asked. It is then possible to distinguish different types of foreign backgrounds, like *Aussiedler*.

More accurate information exists in household surveys where information on parents can be merged with that on an individual (*Mikrozensus* 2005 and 2009, SOEP, Census 2011). For example, in the *Mikrozensus* 2005 data on people living in the same household as their parents, on their parents' country of birth and year of arrival in Germany, and on both current and pre-naturalization citizenship, are available while the *Mikrozensus* 2009 detailed how German nationality was obtained – albeit forming a small sample size mainly of young people. And in SOEP, data on the parents' country of birth, year of arrival in Germany, nationality, language proficiencies and membership of a religious organization are known for those whose parents also participated in the survey.

Overall, then, research on mixed people in Germany is limited because datasets that contain the variables that will allow the identification of mixed people are scarce, albeit growing. Up until German reunification, migrants and their descendents were seen as temporary workers, an out-group in German society. After reunification, the national myth could be challenged by the question of their integration, but without a focus on discrimination. In contrast, research in France currently focuses on both integration and discrimination, with the lack of recognition of migrants and their descendents coming to an end during the 1980s. The question of French national identity, the fight against discrimination and concerns about integration, then became a hot spot of political and scientific debates. We will now consider the processes by which French researchers came to focus on these topics and their impact on the study of mixedness.

France: from integration to the fight against discrimination

For many years French researchers and politicians did not recognize that France was a country of immigration. This is why no criterion other than an individual's current citizenship was available in quantitative surveys, partly hiding people with migration backgrounds and ignoring mixed people. But since the 1990s, quantitative surveys where mixed people could be identified according to various criteria such as parental nationality, country of birth, language or religion (but not ethnicity) were developed.

The French model of integration is based on the principle of equality among French citizens and the non-recognition of any particularism in the public sphere (Schnapper, 1991). Schnapper notes that an individualized integration process is premised on public institutions, such as school, rather than belonging to an ethnic community. The principle of individual citizenship influenced social research in France through the establishment of French sociology by Emile Durkheim. His universalistic and patriotic views strongly influenced French sociologists' lack of awareness of people with a foreign background right up to the 1960s, after which researchers began to study migrants' integration (Schnapper, 1998). This lack of recognition of the French history of immigration is also linked to the issue that 'neither the "ethnic" nor the immigration issue played a role in the birth of [the French] republic' (Noiriel, 1992, p. 69). Noiriel notes that mass foreign migration to France started during the second half of the nineteenth century when the French nation's framework was already in place, with equality and the rejection of any rights based on the origin-forming the roots of the French republic. This historical context explains why nationality became the criterion of social categorization rather than ethnicity.

This history of individualized integration influenced the design of the French Census. The need to count the foreign population and that touched by the reform of the Civil Code on nationality that established a double *jus soli*[2] might explain why a question about nationality was inserted in the French Census from 1851 (Lacroix and Thave, 1997, p. 73). A place of birth question was introduced in 1861. According to Lacroix and Thave (1997), census questions more or less adapt to the evolving nationality code and to the French Empire. In metropolitan France, the census variables have broadly remained the same since 1962. There is no question about an individual's parents other than for cases where they live in the same household. This means that the use of French Censuses to study mixed people is limited. Two surveys based on the French Census give information on parents' nationality and country of birth when both generations were interviewed however: the *Echantillon Démographique Permanent* (EDP)[3] and the *Enquête sur l'Histoire Familiale* from 1999 (EHF).

By the mid-1980s, political debate over the reform of the French nationality code and French national identity highlighted the specific situation of second and third generation 'immigrants'. This debate stemmed from concerns about the rise of the extreme right on one hand and the political mobilization on the nationality of North African people and their children on the other (Weil, 2009, pp. 248–80). Consequently, political institutions to promote integration and knowledge about racism were created, and a need for large-scale datasets to study persons with a migration background was recognized. In 1992, the first quantitative dataset aiming to study the assimilation of first and second generation international migrants in comparison to a representative sample was initiated: the *Mobilité Géographique et Insertion Sociale* survey (MGIS). The previous distinction between national and non-national became replaced by one between immigrants and their descendants.

Direct questions about parental background allowing for the identification of mixed people have become more frequent in French datasets since the 1990s. For example, questions on either the country of birth or the nationality of parents, or both, have been developed for most surveys on education and labour market integration. In the *Education* (1992) and *Panel des élèves* (1995) surveys, both questions were asked simultaneously, while in surveys about labour market integration, the country of birth of the parents not living in the household was asked (*Enquête sur la Formation et la Qualification Professionnelle* since 1993, *Générations* since 1995, *Emploi* survey since 2005), followed by the introduction of a parents' nationality question (*Générations* since 2001, *Emploi* survey since 2005). The introduction of such questions means that it has become possible to study mixed people as defined through the country of birth and/or nationality of their parents. In the MGIS survey for example, mixed people can be identified using the country of birth and current nationality of parents for people who are first or second generation migrants. In parallel, language became a key issue to understanding people's integration during the 1990s (MGIS, *Education*, EHF).

While large-scale datasets where mixed people were able to be identified by their parents' country of birth, nationality and/or language became more common in France from the 1990s, however, the issues remained hotly debated among both politicians and researchers. The use of ethnicity as a social marker in the first analyses of the MGIS survey was the cause of a heated debate. Parallel to methodological criticisms on the definition of people's ethnicity, the French individualized conception of integration[4] was called upon to condemn the use of ethnic categories. The *fichier juif* was also cited in this condemnation – a document initially identified as the Jewish Census made by the police headquarters in Ile-de-France under the Vichy government collaborating with the Third Reich.[5] The discussion about the nature of this document that occurred in the 1990s deeply influenced the French debate on 'ethnic statistics' which then became bound up with a fear of cataloguing and identifying people according to their ethnicity. All of this was used to justify the failure to take account of ethnic origin in official statistics, especially in the national Census. The question of ethnic categories then is highly sensitive in France, as it is in Germany, resulting in an inability for researchers to identify mixed people according to their parents' or their own ethnicity.

By the late 1990s, political discourse had shifted from a focus on the fight against racism to a fight against discrimination. As in Germany, an institutional framework for anti-discrimination policies was implemented gradually, without specifying the 'statistical framework for such action' (Simon, 2007, p. 52). In the scientific arena, the rhetoric of the 1990s had the consequence that the next quantitative survey that over-sampled people with a migration background – *Histoires de vie. Construction des identités* (HDV) – was not conducted until 2003, followed by the *Trajectoires et Origines* (TeO) in 2008. Both surveys included questions on the interviewee's self-identity and feelings of having been discriminated against, but no data was collected about people's ethnic characteristics because of the sensitive nature of the topic. While in the HDV survey, mixed people can be identified on the basis of their parents' place and nationality at birth only, in the TeO, their parents' different nationality, country of birth, migration path, language and/or religion can be used.

In France, as is the case in Germany, mixed people are not defined on the basis of their ethnicity but as people whose parents were socialized in two different countries. Mixed people can then be identified in French data according to the parental nationality and/or place of birth. Further, French large-scale datasets are not precise enough for mother-tongue to be used to identify mixed people. Other than in the *Education* and *Panel des élèves* surveys, questions on parents' language address its transmission to the second generation rather than parental mother-tongue. To identify mixed people according to their parents' socialization, neither the current citizenship of an individual's parents nor their countries of birth are sufficient criteria. Indeed, parents' current nationality does not allow knowledge of whether or not the parents were socialized in different countries. Country of birth is not a sufficient criterion either because it does not distinguish French expatriates and inhabitants of these regions. Indeed, French *rapatriés* (returnees) from the former colonies have other paths of integration and socialization to those available to international migrants and their descendents (Alba and Silberman, 2002). The distinction between the two populations is not insignificant in a context where intermarriage between French *rapatriés* from the former Algerian, Tunisian and Moroccan colonies and French citizens born in France was more likely to occur than between French-born citizens and natives from Maghreb. This is why the TeO survey authors aimed to identify people who have parents of French descent born in the former French colonies or who are French *rapatriés* themselves. Thus it is necessary to have as much information as possible on people's migration path, including the year of arrival of their parents, in order to study mixed people.

Statistical categories follow the trajectories of nationality acts and of political and scientific debates, based on a universalist conception of the French nation and on a fear both of cataloguing people and of the extreme right. As a consequence, the former 'foreigners' category became the category of 'immigrant' of the first, second or third generation. In France and in Germany, researchers mainly are concerned with the integration of people with a foreign background. While the fight against discrimination did not influence the collection of quantitative data on ethnicity in Germany, the issue was raised in France and resulted in the creation of more datasets that over-sampled people with a migration background and increasingly asked questions about discrimination. Even though surveys about discrimination exist in France

(MGIS, HDV and TeO), the fight against discrimination did not result in questions on people's ethnicity which, as I now discuss, is the case in Britain.

Britain: the focus on ethnicity

In contrast to Germany and France, the 'Mixed' category in Britain's datasets is built upon people's ethnicity and 'race'. This is the result of anti-discrimination policies and the fact that the boundary between 'Us' and 'Them' in Britain is not nationality but ethnicity. Indeed, since 2001, a 'Mixed' category has been added to the census question on ethnicity. Mixed people then are identified in large-scale datasets according to their ethnicity rather than their parental migration background.

Historically nationality seems not to have been a major criterion in being considered part of British society. The British Empire and its evolution strongly affected the definition of who is part of the national group and who is not. First, in contrast to the limiting of ethnic categories to non-metropolitan territories during the French Empire, the racial categories used in the British Empire were imported to the UK (Favell, 1998, p. 119). This imperial racial classification was rooted in a justification of the 'English race' and its superiority that had developed from the seventeenth century (Banton, 1977). Second, the British Nationality Act of 1948 confirmed the status of British subject to the Crown in the British Empire without any criterion of national belonging. The distinction between foreigners and British subjects did not map directly onto the one between an ethnic 'Us' and 'Them': 'In absence of a meaningful concept of citizenship, British immigration policy had to operate on a proxy[:] … race' (Joppke, 1999, p. 101). Since the 1960s, the evolution of the definition of British nationality has been shaped by responses to non-white immigration from the New Commonwealth (Hansen, 1999). In this way, the British Empire had an impact on the construction of the 'Other' as non-white people. Thus the border between the in- and the out-group was established around race rather than nationality, even though nationality is interwoven with awareness of ethnic and racial difference. The reform of the Nationality Act of 1981 aimed at juxtaposing British citizenship with immigration law (*ibid.*, p. 111), but the question of who is part of the British nation remains. The identification of mixed people according to their parents' nationality only then seems irrelevant because it does not reflect the connection one parent may have with Britain.

The focus on race rather than nationality was the reason why a strong distinction was made between border control, dealing with international migrants, and race relation policies, focusing on ethnic minorities (Favell, 1998). Rather than thinking of a process of integration through nationality, countering racial discrimination was regarded as a way to create social cohesion in British society. The dominant logic was that 'there would be equality of opportunity, and hence inter-racial harmony, if the one factor that most provokes inter-racial distrust and conflict could be eliminated: racial discrimination' (*ibid.*, p. 116). Race Relations Acts were passed in 1965 and 1968 to this end. Because these first laws concerned direct discrimination, a new act was passed in 1976 to eliminate indirect discrimination. It proposed an administrative framework to achieve this goal, creating the Commission for Racial Inequality (CRE), which was integrated into the Equality and Human Rights Commission under the 2006 Equality Act. Collection of data on ethnicity was seen as a way to fight discrimination: 'As soon as 1978, the government demanded that a question on ethnicity be inserted in the 1981 census with a view to obtaining authoritative and reliable information about ethnic minorities' (Ringelheim, 2006, p. 44). Here, self-identification was seen by the CRE as 'the norm, while other-classification is accepted in limited circumstances' (*ibid.*, p. 47). The identification of mixed people in large-scale datasets was then questioned.

This political context has had a strong impact on social scientific research in Britain. Indeed, there is a split between research on race relations and on nationalism (Schnapper, 1998). Unlike German and French research, in the British case the main focus is on race and racism against ethnic minorities rather than on migration and integration of foreigners and their descendents. The US civil rights movement had a strong impact in this respect, as well as connections between the US and British academic worlds, and the 'heritage of the British Empire' (Schönwälder, 2010, p. 112). Whereas in the 1970s the 'diverse immigrant groups [could] be lumped together into a single class as "coloured people"' (Smith, 1977, p. 331), by the early 1980s minorities were labelled as 'black' and the 'new British population [was described] in terms of a black–white divide' (Modood and Berthoud, 1997, p. 8). Commentators argue that this was due to recession and its stronger impact on ethnic minorities. This 'dualistic approach' has been subject to criticism since the 1990s, although it still has some influence. Ethnicity then, rather than nationality or country of birth, is the major criterion of distinction between ethnic minorities and the majority, and to identify mixed people.

Since the late 1970s, there has been a vigorous debate on how to categorize people according to their ethnicity in large-scale datasets. Numerous articles have been published about ethnic categories and how to identify mixed-race people in such surveys. One criticism of the 1991 Census was that there was no 'Mixed' category. In that Census, mixed people had either to tick one ethnic category only or to write their ethnicity in an 'open response' box, without knowing what the official recoding frames would be (Owen, 2001). The 'Black–Other' and 'Other–Other' categories were constructed to include people who had parents from different ethnic groups. But these categories did not include mixed people only. Besides, people with a mixed ethnic background could have ticked a single category or their open written response could have been recoded under other categories. Significantly then, the 2001 and 2011 Census provided a 'Mixed' box, with sub-categories.

The issue of ethnic categorization in the British Census is of particular relevance since other large-scale datasets adopt its categories, including the

General Household Survey (GHS, merged into the General Lifestyle Survey), the Labour Force Survey (LFS), the Fourth National Survey of Ethnic Minorities, 1994 (FNSEM), the British Household Panel Survey (BHPS, incorporated into the new Understanding Society survey) and the Citizenship Survey (HOCS).[6] The surveys conducted between 1992 and 2000 used the 1991 Census ethnic response categories, and the ones since then have used the 2001 Census format.[7]

The question of ethnicity is so central in Britain that other variables that might be used to identify mixed people often are not asked in large-scale surveys. Notably, a question about parental birthplace was last asked in the 1971 Census. Since then, few quantitative surveys have gathered information on the country of birth of parents who were not interviewed in the survey: the GHS (since 1983), the BHPS (1999–2000, 2008–9), the British Social Attitudes survey (BSA) (2006), and the HOCS (from 2007–8). But, as noted above in relation to France and Germany, country of birth is not sufficient to identify mixed people either. For example, a person could be born in Africa but have an Asian background. Indeed, as Bagley (1972) notes, among marriages between people born in Britain and those who are immigrants, some of these immigrants might be expatriates or their descendents. That is why precise questions about the connection to Africa and Asia were asked in the FNSEM. Further, questions on nationality are uncommon and only concern parents interviewed in the survey (GHS, LFS). One exception is the BSA (1995, 2003), which asked whether or not both parents, the mother or the father were British citizens at an individual's birth. In addition, detailed questions about the religion of parents are asked in some waves of the BSA. Questions on the individual's childhood such as the religion he/she was brought up in (HOCS, 2003, 2010–11) or questions on language most often spoken at home (HOCS 2001, since 2007–8) might be asked, but these allow neither for the identification of people of mixed faith nor of mixed language background.

Household surveys provide detailed information on each member of a household. For example, data on year of arrival in Britain of immigrant parents who live in the same household as their child is collected in the 1971 Census, the GHS and the LFS, as well as parental country of birth (British Census, GHS, LFS, FNSEM, BHPS), parental ethnicity and religion (GHS, LFS, BHPS, Census) and aspects of language proficiencies (Census, BHPS). Thus, as in Germany and France, household surveys allow for some identification of mixed people based on various characteristics.

The concern with fighting ethnic discrimination using data collected in quantitative surveys means that it is difficult to identify mixed people using any other criteria than ethnicity in Britain. Self-identification and ethnic background do not always correspond to each other, however. Indeed, self-identification is shaped by social background, social integration, discrimination, age, gender and so on. Under these circumstances, it may be problematic to conduct research on those defining themselves as 'mixed' or 'other', knowing that it may not strictly fit their ethnic background. If a researcher wishes to identify and study mixed people on the basis of the place of socialization of their parents, as they can do in Germany and France, then they will require data on people's own, and their parents' migration paths as a whole – data that often is not a focus of British large-scale surveys.

Conclusion

This chapter has discussed the ways that, in Germany, France and Britain, conceptions of the 'Us' of the nation and the 'Them' outside it are two sides of the same coin, interlocked in political, media and academic debates, and shaping the data that is collected in large-scale surveys. Germany and France started with a 'foreigner' category that developed into a 'people with migration background' category, while Britain has focused on 'ethnic minorities'. The various visions of social cohesion in these countries influenced social scientific research and the study of mixed people using quantitative surveys.

Large-scale datasets, then, are strongly influenced by the national context in which they are produced. A nation's conceptions, collective memory, nationality acts, social cohesion, policies (e.g. against discrimination), and political and academic debates, are intertwined. The interplay of this range of factors may be a process in common, but how they influence each other and the consequences of their interaction for the data collected in large-scale surveys is – as we have seen for Germany, France and Britain – quite different in each context.

But if statistics are the product of national conceptions, policy orientations and so on, they are also 'to bodies and social types what maps are to territories: they flatten and enclose' (Appadurai, 1993, p. 334). Through the generation of categories that serve as borders around groups considered to have a common identity, statistics create the divisions between 'Us' and 'Them' and build our social reality. The use of categories in large-scale datasets then, is not neutral. The creation of categories is the product of political and scientific debate. In turn, these categories have an impact on society. The criteria used to define mixed people in large-scale datasets influence the conceptualization and social reality of who is considered 'mixed' and who is not.

A person can be defined as 'mixed' either because his or her parents are seen as coming from two different groups, each having a different nation, culture, language, religion and so on, or because that person defines him- or herself as mixed. Currently, this latter definition is used in Britain, but not in Germany or France. In Britain, mixed people can indeed be identified mainly through their ethnic self-identification but in some surveys according to other criteria like the country of birth. And in Germany, quantitative surveys where it is possible to identify mixed people are still scarce but increasing and becoming more detailed. The current nationality of the parents is indeed the most common criteria to identify them, but the country of birth and migration status are starting to be asked. In France too, criteria to identify mixed people in large-scale surveys are increasing. While questions on the parents' nationality, country of birth and language started to be asked in the 1990s, the detailed migration status of parents has latterly begun to be asked too. Under these circumstances, for researchers who wish to undertake an international comparison of mixed people, criteria other than ethnicity have to be used. The capacity to compare the numbers and situation of mixed people in different countries is dependent not only on the substantive focus of research interests but also on the possibilities for identifying and enumerating mixed people in large-scale surveys.

Notes

1 SOEP, as well as other surveys in France – the EDP for example – and Britain – the GLF since 2005 and the BHPS – are household longitudinal surveys. The availability of information on parents once living in the same household as the individual and interviewed in the survey enables researchers to identify mixed people.
2 In countries following the *jus soli*, citizenship is dependent on place of birth. 'Double *jus soli*' means that an individual having foreign parents will become a citizen of his/her country of birth if his/her parents were born in that country themselves.
3 The EDP provides information about the country of birth of an individual's parents and the parents' nationality at the time of the person's birth. The past citizenship of the parent is known only if the person became a French citizen when he/she was under 18 thanks to parental naturalization. Other than these people, mixed people can be studied using the EDP only by looking at their parents' country of birth and current nationality.
4 Equality before law and no distinction between French citizens on the basis on their origin, race or religion was stated in article 1 of the Constitution of the Fifth Republic of 1958.
5 In fact, the document was a set of files of arrested and deported Jews produced afterwards.
6 The British Social Attitudes Survey is one of the exceptions.
7 The BHPS included the 2001 Census categories in 2003–4.

References

Alba, R. and Silberman, R. (2002) 'Decolonization Immigrations and the Social Origins of the Second Generation: The Case of North Africans in France', *International Migration Review*, 36 (4): 1169–93.

Anderson, B. (2006 [1991]) *Imagined Communities: Reflections on the Origin and Spread of Nationalism*, New York: Verso.

Appadurai, A. (1993) 'Number in the Colonial Imagination', in C.A. Breckenridge and P. Van Der Veer (eds), *Orientalism and the Postcolonial Predicament*, Philadelphia, PA: University of Pennsylvania Press.

Bagley, C. (1972) 'Patterns of Inter-Ethnic Marriage in Great Britain', *Phylon*, 33 (4): 373–79.

Banton, M. (1977) *The Idea of Race*, Cambridge: Cambridge University Press.

Bommes, M. (2010) 'Migration Research in Germany: The Emergence of a Generalised Research Field in a Reluctant Immigration Country', in D. Thränhardt and M. Bommes (eds), *National Paradigms of Migration Research*, IMIS, 13, Göttingen: V&R unipress, Osnabrück: Universitätsverlag Osnabrück.

EFFNATIS (European Forum for Migration Studies) (2001) *Effectiveness of National Integration Strategies Towards Second Generation Migrant Youth in a Comparative European Perspective* – EFFNATIS, http://www.efms.uni-bamberg.de/pdf/finalreportk.pdf (accessed 6 January 2012).

Favell, A. (1998) *Philosophies of Integration: Immigration and the Idea of Citizenship in France and Britain*, London: Macmillan Press.

Green, S. (1999) 'La politique de la nationalité en Allemagne: La prédominance de l'appartenance ethnique sur la résidence', in P. Weil and R. Hansen (eds), *Nationalité et citoyenneté en Europe*, Paris: Editions La Découverte.

Hansen, R. (1999) 'Le droit de l'immigration et de la nationalité au Royaume-Uni: Des sujets aux citoyens', in P. Weil and R. Hansen (eds), *Nationalité et citoyenneté en Europe*, Paris: Editions La Découverte.

Haug, S. (2004) 'Soziale Integration durch soziale Einbettung in Familie, Verwandtschafts-und Freundesnetzwerke', *Zeitschrift für Bevölkerungswissenschaft*, 29 (2): 163–92.

Joppke, C. (1999) *Immigration and the Nation-State: The United States, Germany, and Great Britain*, Oxford: Oxford University Press.

——(2000) 'Mobilisation of Culture and the Reform of Citizenship Law: Germany and the United States', in R. Koopmans and P. Statham (eds), *Challenging Immigration and Ethnic Relations Politics: Comparative European Perspectives*, Oxford: Oxford University Press.

Klekowski von Koppenfels, A. (2009) 'From German to Migrants: Aussiedler Migration to Germany', in T. Tsuda (ed.), *Diasporic Homecomings: Ethnic Return Migration in Comparative Perspective*, Stanford, CA: Stanford University Press.

Labbé, M. (1998) '"Race" et "Nationalité" dans les recensements du Troisième Reich. De l'auto-déclaration au diagnostic racial', *Histoire et mesure*, 13 (1–2): 195–223.

Lacroix, J. and Thave, S. (1997) 'Les immigrés dans les recensements: décalages entre législation et outils de mesure', *Revue française des affaires sociales*, 51 (2): 71–99.

Merton, R.K. (1964) 'Intermarriage and Social Structure: Fact and Theory', in R.L. Coser (ed.), *In the Family: Its Structure and Functions*, New York: St Martin's Press.

Modood, T. and Berthoud, R. (eds) (1997) *Ethnic Minorities in Britain: Diversity and Disadvantage*, London: Policy Studies Institute.

Noiriel, G. (1992) 'Difficulties in French Historical Research on Immigration', in D.L. Horowitz and G. Noiriel (eds), *Immigrants in Two Democracies: French and American Experience*, New York: New York University Press.

Owen, C. (2001) '"Mixed Race" in Official Statistics', in D. Parker and M. Song (eds), *Rethinking 'Mixed Race'*, London: Pluto Press.

Ringelheim, J. (2006) *Processing Data on Racial or Ethnic Origin for Antidiscrimination Policies: How to Reconcile the Promotion of Equality with the Right to Privacy?* Center for Human Rights and Global Justice Working Paper, 13.

Schnapper, D. (1991) *La France de l'intégration: Sociologie de la nation en 1990*, Paris: Editions Gallimard.

——(1998) *La relation à l'Autre: Au coeur de la pensée sociologique*, Paris: Editions Gallimard.

Schönwälder, K. (2010) 'Beyond the Race Relations Model: Old Patterns and New Trends in Britain', in D. Thränhardt and M. Bommes (eds), *National Paradigms of Migration Research*, IMIS, 13, Göttingen: V&R unipress, Osnabrück: Universitätsverlag Osnabrück.

Simon, P. (2007) *'Ethnic' Statistics and Data Protection in the Council of Europe Countries Study Report*, Council of Europe, European Commission Against Racism and Intolerance.

Smith, D.J. (1977) *Racial Disadvantage in Britain: The PEP Report*, Harmondsworth: Penguin.

Weil, P. (2009) *Qu'est-ce qu'un Français? Histoire de la nationalité française depuis la Révolution*, Paris: Editions Gallimard.

11 Not the same difference

Notes on mixed-race methodologies

Minelle Mahtani

This chapter will address some methodological challenges I have faced while conducting research in mixed-race studies, paying particular attention to the use of interviews as a way of acquiring information about mixed-race experiences. While we have witnessed the publication of important new work analyzing novels, drama, and art installations on multiraciality (Elam 2011; McNeil 2010), media representations of multiracial people (Squires 2007), tabulating the diverse voices and stories of mixed-race people (De Rango-Adem and Thompson 2010; Hill 2001; O'Hearn 1998; Funderburg 1994) and the critical evaluation of the ontology and epistemology of critical mixed-race studies (Rockquemore, Brunsma and Delgado 2009; Sexton 2008; Spencer 2011), much research in contemporary mixed-race analysis in the social sciences has relied on relatively small samples of open-ended, qualitative interviews. Rockquemore, Brunsma and Delgado (2009: 20) note that:

> the past 10 years of research on the multiracial population has been marked by a move from reliance on case studies, observation of multiracial support groups, and small-scale interview studies, to a broader and more robust stage of data collection and analysis.

In paying attention to the former (small-scale interview studies), rather than the latter sphere, this chapter raises fundamental questions regarding the limitations of the interview in the research process. What difference does it make if a person who identifies as mixed race conducts the interview? What kinds of hierarchical assumptions and racial logics are understood as normative in the research process? What constitutes an insider position in critical mixed-race research? And finally, how might one's own subconscious desires and experiences influence the stories we feel compelled to tell in critical mixed-race theory?

While we have rehearsed similar but not identical arguments in feminist theory along the lines of gender, it is useful to consider the role that one's own identification as a mixed-race researcher plays in altering the methodological terrain in mixed-race studies (see Ali 2006). In this chapter, I examine the epistemological foundations shaping understandings of the relationship between researcher and researched in qualitative analyses in mixed-race studies, and examine my complex and often times complicit position as a woman who identifies as mixed race. I suggest how not only my racialized identity, but also my identity as an upper-middle-class Canadian woman working in the field of journalism influenced the gathering and the analysis of interviews. I draw on my own (now tattered) research diaries in which I have jotted down notes and ideas over the years about the mixed-race research process. I will conclude with some suggestions on how we might attempt efforts at greater transparency and reflexivity as we move forward in critical mixed-race studies.

Before I launch into a critical analysis of the research process I employed (see Mahtani 2002a, 2002b, 2002c), it is useful to delineate my methodological approach. I conducted 24 open-ended, qualitative interviews with self-identified women of mixed-race identity. If they chose to identify as either mixed race, multiracial, or multiethnic, I was interested in speaking to them. I sought out women through word-of-mouth and the posting of signs. The interviews ranged from lasting an hour to four hours, and I recorded all interviews. Because I chose women who self-identified as mixed race, I encountered various methodological dilemmas. This approach was not without its limitations. I had several women volunteer for the study, explaining that they saw themselves as "half Finnish, half French" for example, and that they steadfastly identified as multiethnic – and why wouldn't I interview them? In choosing women to interview in this study, I had to re-examine my recruitment process, and reconsider how it is that I, and subsequently potential participants, conceptualized understandings of both race and ethnicity. In the Canadian context, race and ethnicity are often conflated, and these women saw themselves as mixed race perhaps because they were influenced by perceptions of race as sanctioned through the state-sponsored project of Canadian multicultural policy. I also think it is valuable to note that the women I recruited identified as mostly middle to upper class. This status influenced the commentary I elicited from participants significantly, an issue I address in some of my previous studies (see Mahtani 2002c). I begin by exploring my own stance as a mixed-race woman interviewing other mixed-race women.

Problematizing the insider/outsider dualism in mixed-race studies

Despite the prevalence of qualitative and quantitative analyses concerned with the impact race has on individuals' lives, there remain few studies questioning the role that a scholar's own racial background plays in influencing the analytical lens. Although the anthology *Racing Research, Researching Race* (Twine and Warren 2000) unveiled important methodological dilemmas inherent in conducting research in critical race studies, there still are few analyses that meditate upon the racialized subject positions of both the researcher and researched in mixed-race studies (although see Ali, 2006).

I begin this chapter by interrogating the metaphor of the insider/outsider dualism that so often structures discussions about the interviewing process. Feminist researchers have emphasized the value of greater reflexivity in the research process to challenge myths of objectivity, impartiality and value-free knowledge production (see Oakley 1981). Han suggests that "feminist scholarship has fostered a model based on a sympathetic, egalitarian research process, [distinguishable] by authenticity, reciprocity and intersubjectivity between the researcher and her 'subjects'" (Han 2010: 13). Others, like Gill Valentine, encourage us to complicate the division between researcher and researched, often constituted through the insider/outsider domain. She states:

> researchers who share the same identities with their informants ... are positioned as "insiders" and as such have truer access to knowledge, and a closer, more direct connection with their informants than those who are "outsiders." Underlying this notion of being an "insider" is the assumption that they can somehow produce a more correct interpretation of informants' responses. In contrast, "outsiders" are assumed to have more cultural baggage to deal with.
>
> (Valentine 2002: 117)

How does the presumption of a shared mixed-race identity work to construe an insider and outsider position? I turn to my own experiences to explore this question. During the research process, there were certainly times when my own status as a mixed-race woman of Indian and Iranian descent did foster dialogue. At moments, I discovered that my own mixed-race identity may have helped diminish the fears of participants who were wary of my reasons for carrying out this study. I became very familiar with the phrase, "Oh, you're mixed too? Oh well, then I'll definitely be interviewed!" During a pivotal point in our interview, one participant explained to me how she felt comfortable talking to me as a woman of mixed race:

> You see that's the sort of thing, that I don't necessarily think that I would be able to describe to somebody who wasn't, and I'm going to say it again, I mean you need it for description's sake, but who wasn't of mixed race. I don't think they'd really get it.

I would feel a kinship with a woman because she felt I understood the customs and practices of her Sindi culture, because I identified as Sindi, too. Yet at other times, a woman of partial Iranian descent would giggle with me over an incident that occurred at a Nawrooz (Iranian New Year) party. However, at the same time, I was well aware that my own identification as a woman of mixed race played other roles in the interview process. For example, peppered through many interviews emerged the phrase, "You know what I mean, Minelle" followed by a knowing glance or smile. This sort of shared complicity may have created a more comfortable space for these women to tell their stories – but also prevented them from divulging further detail, given that they simply thought that I "understood" what they were not saying (see also Edwards 1990).

Feminists have long pointed out that there is no single analytical category of "woman" and similarly but not identically, the category of mixed race tends to further obscure the disparate heterogeneous diversity contained within that label. One of the most important findings in my study was that the group of women who were interviewed displayed remarkably different perceptions, beliefs, and experiences of both race and racism (see Mahtani 2002c). As a woman identifying as mixed race, I indeed share commonality with the women I interviewed and at times assume this core basis of unity with them, but it is important to question the expectation for "mutual recognition" among these women who had very different life experiences and who held very different, often opposing, perspectives. Consequently, it is erroneous to assume all mixed-race women are sisters; having "unified subjectivities of shared consciousness through gender" (Gilbert 1994: 92). Light skin privilege and class status, among other factors, also inform important bases for evolving and shifting identifications of "mixed race." Some participants in my study experienced very different kinds of racisms based upon day-to-day decisions made by others regarding their phenotypes. Some of the women experienced racism daily; others, not at all because of white skin privilege and class standing, as mentioned earlier, among other factors. I was separated from many of the women I interviewed through a variety of social cleavages which structure life worlds, like life partner choices, sexual orientation, political activism, age, whether they were adopted or not, outgoing or shy, among countless other salient divisions. While I shared many subject positions with informants, only one of these axes was my own identity as a multiracial person. Ali (2006) notes, in relation to her own experience conducting research in mixed-race studies: "I both identified and disidentified with Josey [a participant in her study] throughout, and this was raced, gendered and classed" (Ali 2006: 481). Doing this research, it became increasingly clear to me that the insider/outsider dualism was simply not a useful metaphor through which to understand my experiences. The boundary between myself and the interviewee was rarely stable and often porous, and I draw from Mullings, who insists that we pay greater attention to the "situated knowledge of both parties in the interview encounter, [and how it] engender[s] a level of trust and co-operation" (Mullings 1999: 4). She suggests it may be more productive to consider "shared spaces" that are not informed by identity-based differences because identities based only on markers such as gender, race and class are not necessarily "fail-safe indicators of an individual's positionality" (ibid.).

One aspect of shared knowing emerging between me and interviewees was not that of a traditional identity marker, but our joint participation in journalism. While conducting interviews, I was employed as a television news producer. As such, I conducted at least three interviews a day (mostly by phone, but some in person), booked guests and prepared hosts for a daily news/current affairs program. My experience as a TV producer and the news angle that I developed in my profession (along with the training courses I took towards improving my news interviewing skills) influenced the ways I conducted interviews with women of mixed race. In particular, interviewing women for this study made me confront issues of my own personality and professional training. My own positioning as a television journalist played a role in the acquisition of data. I was read as a bona-fide journalist by some of the participants in this study, which lent me a credence I was not aware of at the time. Some of the younger interviewees would ask me anxiously afterwards for tips on how to get into journalism. At the same time, many of the women I did end up interviewing worked in journalism too, and many of our conversations reflected our joint interest in this profession where an alliance was temporarily forged based neither upon the social cleavages of ethnicity nor gender, but our experiences in journalism, as the following excerpt from my research diary will show:

> I am sitting in the board room at the network with Emma, where after several attempts, we're finally meeting to conduct this interview. Emma works crazy hours in TV, and it's rare that she knows what her days are like – last time we scheduled, the premier announced a live press conference that day and we had to cancel. But finally, we've managed to find a spare moment to conduct the interview. Emma and I have worked together very sparingly in the past – I might have handed a tape to her or called her about a special. But we've never actually talked. Now, we're half-way through the interview, and she says to me, "You know, I really think mixed-race women occupy a postmodern space." I look at her and smile to myself, thinking excitedly, "Oh my God – there's the clip!" – the sound bite I'm always searching for when conducting my TV interviews. Almost as if reading my mind, Emma grins and says, "Isn't that a great clip?" We both laugh, as if conspiring together.
>
> (Research diary note)

Emma and I shared a moment through our similar experiences working in television, where in the workplace we are constantly searching for "the perfect clip." This may have had an impact upon what Emma chose to reveal during the course of the interview. She no doubt wanted to give what she thought would be good interview, in TV terms (shorter, quippier commentary) and this desire may have influenced the acquisition of the data I received. Clearly, the motivations behind the desire to create shared commonalities among women are diverse. In these situations, I felt I developed a keen rapport with participants based upon our joint interest in the media, rather than upon the more socially prevalent axes of gender or ethnicity. If critical mixed-race theory is going to work to challenge exclusionary tendencies, we must reflexively look at the assumptions and stereotypes as well as our own complex identities that we bring to the field.

The limitations of focusing on the individual experience in critical mixed-race studies

In an important article, Rockquemore, Brunsma and Delgado (2009) delineate several epistemological shifts in mixed-race studies. I will focus my interests on two stages they outline: the problem approach and the variant approach. They assert the problem approach

> emerged out of Jim Crow segregation and focused its inquiry on the confusion and tragedy inherent in being located between two races. From that perspective, marginality was the inevitable destination for mixed-race people. As such, researchers asked questions that reinforced segregation and the structure of Jim Crow and constructed mixed-race people as both barometer and scapegoat by denying them agency.
>
> (Rockquemore, Brunsma and Delgado 2009: 24)

The next stage they discuss is the variant approach, which

> emerg[ed] in the post-Civil Rights era, [and demonstrated] similar epistemological problems coupled with a class bias and a flair for identity politics. It overemphasized the agency of mixed-race people (particularly those that self-identify as multiracial), ignoring structure in favor of an individualistic stance that contained a palpable disdain for Blackness and an eye toward Whiteness.
>
> (ibid.)

I want to focus on Rockquemore, Brunsma and Delgado's suggestion that research that falls within the parameters of the variant approach overemphasizes an individualistic stance. What are the dangers of adopting an individualistic stance in mixed-race studies? To engage with this question, I briefly explore responses online to Maria Root's "Bill of Rights for Racially Mixed People." No researcher in this field will be unfamiliar with Maria Root's Bill of Rights, which cheerfully proclaims mixed-race people's individual right to self-identify. Some of the proclamations in the Bill of Rights include: "I have the right to identify myself differently than my brothers and sisters, I have the right not to be responsible for people's discomfort with my physical ambiguity, I have the right to identify myself differently in different situations, and I have the right to have loyalties and identify with more than one group of people" (Root 1996: 7). The Bill of Rights has received international attention and acclaim. Online, the Bill is celebrated, especially among mothers who see it as a powerful way to shatter stereotypes about their mixed-race children. For example, on the website Circle of Moms:

Motherhood Shared and Simplified, mothers of mixed-race children exuberantly post exclamations of excitement upon discovering the Bill of Rights. A few excerpts from the website include:

> WOWWwww … I LOVE [THE BILL OF RIGHTS]!!!! My 15 yr old biracial son would love that! He is going thru some identity issues around being african american/german/russian american; although, he looks egyptian, mexian, because of the texture of his hair and his color. People give him a bad time about his heritage. They question him all the time. I understand the BILL OF RIGHTS for people of Mixed Heritage.
>
> (http://www.circleofmoms.com/moms-of-bi-racial-babieschildren/bill-of-rights-for-people-of-mixed-heritage-maria-p-root-phd-442161, retrieved April 20 2011)

Another mother exclaims, "I think [sic] it should be posted on BUSES in Malls, create a FLIER for this. Send it all over the world. This empowers our children to stand up for who they are." Yet another mother delights, "Love this!!! I'm going to print this out and put it on the fridge :)"

It appears that the mothers on this website find the Bill of Rights to be particularly compelling. However, the Bill of Rights has been hotly critiqued by scholars like Jared Sexton, who claim that the Bill ensures that mixed race can achieve "distance and distinction from racial blackness" and "disregard[s] … hard-won juridical gains monitored by the civil rights establishment and an obligatory disdain for any future black activity" (Sexton 2008: 77). I am sympathetic to Sexton's claims. The Bill can effectively allow for some mixed-race people to eschew blackness. While announcing one's right to identify any way one chooses is admirable, the structural and material reality of racism (not to mention the historical and geographical legacies of racial privilege and marginalization) dictate that if one is perceived as black, self-proclamations like, "Oh no, I'm not black, I'm actually mixed race!" will not do much to insulate one from racist acts. To put it another way: the manifesto is not an anti-racist security blanket.

Michele Elam points out the challenges of self-identifying as mixed race through her cogent analysis of Aaron McGruder's comic strip *The Boondocks*, which features a biracial girl named Jazmine Dubois. In the comic strip, Jazmine's black father, Tom, and her white mother, Sarah, are both attorneys (read: insulated by socio-economic class privilege). Jazmine is light skinned and is quick to assert that she is definitely not black, but mixed race, stamping her foot angrily, insisting that she "resents racial categories!" (quoted in Elam 2011: 64). She regularly faces contempt from her playmate Huey, who identifies as black, and he showers Jazmine with disdain, claiming that she is simply suffering from a kind of racial delusion. Elam sees *The Boondocks* as a kind of popular cultural intervention into contemporary conversations about multiraciality. Through the example of Jazmine's efforts to proclaim her multiracial identity, Elam illustrates how race is often problematically portrayed among mixed-race advocates as an issue of free will (Elam 2011). Keeping Elam's commentary in mind, it is worthwhile to return to the Bill of Rights and ask why it is that the Bill has sparked such enthusiasm among the mothers of mixed-race children on the webpage cited earlier. The desire to enshrine the Bill of Rights on their refrigerators, for example, certainly indicates that the Bill has struck a chord. The Bill of Rights' popularity is in part due to its optimistic nature and declarative tone. But I would caution parents from seeing it as a fool-proof strategy to challenge racism, because the Bill can conveniently evacuate race from the conversation, depoliticizing the very real material consequences of unequal power differentials between racialized groups. What the Bill of Rights can do is cement a disturbing neoliberal belief among some parents of mixed-race children that their kids can simply choose to identify any way they want, without necessarily preparing their children for the potential racist onslaught that can follow.

I have paid particular attention to the intellectual controversy surrounding the Bill of Rights not because it is my goal to critique Maria Root's laudatory attempts to offer mixed-race people, as she puts it, a "set of affirmations or 'rights' as reminders to break the spell of the delusion that creates race to the detriment of us all" (Root 1996: 6). I believe that Root's goals in penning the Bill of Rights must be located within a particular geographical and historical context, in which I see Root as responding directly to the "problem approach" that shaped the pervasive psychopathology surrounding the mixed-race experience. Mixed-race interventions like Root's must be situated within a constellation of historical and geographical matrices, paying particular attention to the precise historical moment, intellectual valence, and political climate in which it was produced (indeed, Root notes that the chapter which includes the original version of the Bill of Rights emerged through an invitation to give a keynote address to the University of California at Santa Barbara's student group, Variations, for a conference on multiraciality in 1994). One also cannot forget that Root's approach to multiraciality emerges from her own training and experience as a successful psychologist, and I would argue that within the realm of psychology there has been much greater emphasis on encouraging individuals to deal with identity questions "one-on-one" by changing themselves, rather than necessarily offering them avenues towards challenging structural injustices. My point is to show how the Bill of Rights' focus on agency and freedom of choice echoes a disturbing tendency in multiracial research to focus on the individual's experience of race, rather than exploring how a mixed-race identity shapes and is in turn shaped by ongoing patterns of systemic racism. What sorts of methodological approaches can we develop that will get at some of those complicated issues?

The interview process

Lastly, I want to pay attention to the role of the interview in the mixed-race research process. Although I initially planned to engage in one-way interviews, I soon discovered that the process took on less of a question–answer format and more the form of an exchange during moments in the interview. I felt some responsibility to discuss my own mixed-race experiences with these women, given the seeming therapeutic atmosphere I was creating for them to divulge these deeply personal stories. Confiding such personal matters established a level of personal involvement which I did not want to ignore. I found myself engaged in conversation at points during the interview because I wanted to establish a rapport between us. In many ways, although this seems like a facetious comparison, the interviews felt like twenty-four blind dates. I cringed when I saw any interviewee ill at ease and wanted to reassure her, especially since I likened the interview process to an emotional excavation given the intensely personal experiences which are revealed. During some of the interviews, the women would become increasingly emotional, and even shed a tear or two. I want to cite a fairly long passage from one of my interviews, where we lapsed into dialogue during one section of the interview:

MAKEDA: So where were we? Oh yes, I was dissing my ex-boyfriend!

MINELLE: But you're so good at it! (shared laughter) It's just funny to hear you talk, in some ways, so much of what you talk about, is stuff that comes up for me. About whiteness. I mean I've felt similarly about not dating white men anymore, and then I go and date another white man!

MAKEDA: Yeah, especially if you declare a moratorium! (shared laughter)

MINELLE: And it's so ironic, and I know I'm lying. I don't think desire works that way. I don't think you can limit it, as much as you try.

MAKEDA: No, you're right, you might find yourself in a situation where, which doesn't transcend race, but might bring you closer in a way? That you haven't found with other people? This relationship I have with people who I've been close to, on an intellectual basis? Like in terms of school, and mentors, and like, that whole thing is really complicated to me, too. Like who I think of being a voice of knowledge. You know? So that to me has been a big issue, like where is knowledge? And these aren't new questions, like Dr. [X] and her work has talked about. She's talked about being a professor … that's another interesting thing. Is when you find out there's a time when these same women of color who have [spoken about these issues], and you find out, "Oh, but she's with a white man!" You know? Like I remember hearing that about her, and it's like, "Oh she's with a white man … "

MINELLE: I know, it's like: how can she preach all this while at home, while in her personal life …

MAKEDA: I KNOW! And a lot of people have said that about people at school, too. Like [X], or whatever. It's so funny!

MINELLE: In terms of battling their own demons, and then they have all these people talking about them …

MAKEDA: I think sometimes, what frustrates me is that I'm the only person who ever thinks about these things in relation to this desire? But it's not

> true, when I'm around YOU, or whoever, they are completely normal questions to be asking? Or just ah, and it cuts both ways, the idea of wanting to be, liked and loved for our difference, and not be, and at the same time not to have that difference to be made absolute? But that it somehow, is a clearly defining, quality?

There are many avenues through which I can dissect this interview excerpt. Much is divulged and I have changed some identifying information to ensure anonymity. However, in this excerpt, I want to focus on the rapport between us. While some may read my interjections as leading, I suggest that it offered an opportunity for me to clarify the thoughts of the interviewee. In this situation, Makeda elucidated the notion of transcending racial divides. This resulted, for me, in the acquisition of very rich information. We then embarked upon another shared axes – our joint impressions of professors at college – at which point Makeda extended that it seemed perfectly natural, in her words, to talk about these issues (of race and power and academic prestige) with me. Joining in conversation with her, I believe, facilitated her comfort level during the interview process, just as it facilitated my own comfort level, which cannot be overlooked. Although one might read my interjections as a way of tainting data, I suggest that in fact this exchange is much more natural than remaining mute. My own silence during an interview would still play a major part in the association between the interviewee and researcher. Even the most basic "yes" – a simple affirmative utterance – is inherently laden with all sorts of powerful effects because of its extraverbal content. Any exchange between two people – regardless of an interview or a dialogue – provides an immensely complex context in which meaning is produced and contested. As I remind my journalism students regularly, it is virtually impossible to carry out an objective interview. Any exchange is a loaded one as every communication establishes a relationship, or a cocoon, between individuals. By continuing to insist upon our own unbiased status, or assuming we can adopt this stance, we are in fact ignoring the very real baggage we bring to each interview and the potential impacts of the content of this baggage. If I attempted to veil these experiences, I very well may have created a situation which is highly artificial, heightening the tensions between the researcher and interviewee. In our day-to-day interactions, we rarely engage in pointed, one-way dialogue, and given the intensely personal nature of these interviews, I found it difficult, and unfair, to stay silent.

To end, I will share one last research vignette:

> I am at home, eating macaroni and cheese in the company of my best friend from work. She's always been interested in my interviews and asks me how my interview with Emma has gone. Taking a sip of red wine, I reflect for a moment before I answer the question. My friend knows Emma intimately on both a personal and professional level, but I'm well aware that the interview is confidential. I say guardedly, "Well, she told

> me a lot about her Dad in Malaysia," thinking that wasn't divulging a great deal. Anita looks at me strangely. "That's odd. Her Dad died a year ago. Did she tell you that?" I'm stunned because Emma referred to her father all the way through the interview as if he was alive. I change the subject, but my mind is whirring. Just how much did Emma tell me, and did she in fact keep other important details from me knowing that I am her work colleague and she wants to guard her privacy?
>
> (Research diary note)

I want to mark the very real dangers of attributing an absolute value to the gathered narratives. I do not want to suggest that the story is all that there is – the telling and reading of the narratives is always grounded in particular social processes that can go beyond the stories. These interviews reveal the limitations of acquiring the story – certain reflections can only be told at particular social moments. My own participation in these interviews played a role in the acquiring of data, where I performed multiple roles, expressing compassion and sympathy at different times. These stories do not at all begin to capture the ways in which the body narrates the experience of multiraciality. This particular scenario details my concern that there is often so much that is not being expressed due to the limits and constraints of the interview process. Of course, it is almost trite to say that no story told through an interview is ever complete. Stories as expressed through the interview process are always subjective, revealing some of the interviewee's experience, but of course, not all. We narrate tales of our experiences in particular, partial ways, re-working them, shaping them over time, and moving and modifying them after reflecting upon our moods, the place, and the time of the interview. There is a constant process of readjusting our stories to be aligned with the very time and place, not to mention listener, of the tale. Like the diverse, active, and embodied lives of the women I interviewed and their subsequent discussion of their multiple identities, we must acknowledge the multiple ways we can tell those layered stories and how our telling is altered dependent upon a variety of contexts. These narratives may be re-envisioned as re-assemblings of pastiches, bits and (sound) bites reflecting an incessant playfulness within the re-tellings of a life story. In this brief chapter, I have tried to offer a self-reflexive analysis of my own role in conducting interviews with mixed-race women. Ali, in reflecting upon her experience conducting research on multiraciality, concludes that she might have conducted her own research differently in hindsight, but that "even small changes would inevitably mean that it would have been a different piece of research, not necessarily a better piece of research" (Ali 2006: 482). I have asserted that there are many ways of telling the story of a racialized and gendered existence, and in the analysis, a plethora of possibilities pervade. Critical mixed-race researchers may benefit from dissecting the assumptions we make about the shared differences with those who we study, what role we play in the acquisition of research on multiracial people, and finally, how we choose to present these stories, towards becoming more transparent about potentially complicit desires, experiences and beliefs as we go about conducing research in mixed-race studies.

References

Ali, Suki. 2006. "Racializing Research: Managing Power and Politics?" *Ethnic and Racial Studies* 29 (3): 471–86.

Caballero, Chamion, Jo Haynes and Leon Tikly. 2007. "Researching Mixed Race in Education: Perceptions, Policies and Practices" *Race, Ethnicity and Education* 10 (3): 345–62.

DaCosta, Kimberly McClain. 2007. *Making Multiracials: State, Family and Market in the Redrawing of the Color Line*. Stanford, CA: Stanford University Press.

De Rango-Adem, A. and Andrea Thompson (eds). 2010. *Other Tongues: Mixed-Race Women Speak Out*. Toronto: Inanna Publications and Education Inc.

Edwards, Rosalind. 1990. "Connecting Method and Epistemology: A White Woman Interviewing Black Women" *Women's Studies International Forum* 13: 477–90.

Elam, Michele. 2011. *The Souls of Mixed Folk: Race, Politics and Aesthetics in the New Millennium*, Stanford, CA: Stanford University Press.

Funderburg, Lise. 1994. *Black, White, Other: Biracial Americans Talk about Race and Identity*, New York: William Morrow and Company, Inc.

Gilbert, Melissa. 1994. "The Politics of Location: Doing Feminist Research at 'Home'" *Professional Geographer* 46 (1): 90–96.

Han, Judy. 2010. "Neither Friends nor Foes: Thoughts on Ethnographic Distance" *Geoforum* 41 (1): 11–14.

Hill, Lawrence. 2001. *Black Berry, Sweet Juice: On Being Black and White in Canada*, Toronto: HarperCollins.

Kaufman, Barry. 1991. *Happiness is a Choice*. New York: Fawcett.

McNeil, Daniel. 2010. *Sex and Race in the Black Atlantic*. London: Routledge.

Mahtani, Minelle. 2002a. "What's in a Name? Exploring the Employment of 'Mixed Race' as an Ethno-Racial Identification" *Ethnicities* 2 (4): 469–90.

——2002b. "Tricking the Border Guards: Performing Race" *Environment and Planning D: Society and Space* 20: 425–40.

——2002c. "Interrogating the Hyphen-Nation: Canadian Multicultural Policy and 'Mixed Race' Identities" *Social Identities: Journal for the Study of Race, Nation and Culture* 8 (1): 67–90.

Mullings, Beverley. 1999. "Insider or Outsider, Both or Neither: Some Dilemmas of Interviewing in a Cross-Cultural Setting" *Geoforum* 30: 337–50.

Oakley, Ann. 1981. "Interviewing Women: A Contradiction in Terms" in H. Roberts (ed.). *Doing Feminist Research*. London: RKP Press, 30–61.

O'Hearn, Clandine Chiawei (ed.) 1998. *Half and Half: Writers on Growing Up Biracial and Bicultural*. New York: Pantheon.

Rockquemore, Kerry Ann, David Brunsma and Daniel Delgado. 2009. "Racing to Theory or Retheorizing Race? Understanding the Struggle to Build a Multiracial Identity Theory" *Journal of Social Issues* 65 (1): 13–34.

Root, Maria. 1996. "A Bill of Rights for Racially Mixed People" in Maria Root (ed.). *The Multiracial Experience: Racial Borders as the New Frontier*. London: Sage. 3–14.

Senna, Danzy. 1998. "The Mulatto Millennium" in Claudine Chiawei O'Hearn (ed.). *Half and Half: Writers on Growing Up Biracial and Bicultural.* New York: Pantheon, 12–27.

Sexton, Jared. 2008. *Amalgamation Schemes: Antiblackness and the Critique of Multiracialism.* Minneapolis, MN: University of Minnesota Press.

Spencer, Rainier. 2011. *Reproducing Race: The Paradox of Generation Mix.* Boulder, CO: Lynne Rienner Publishers.

Squires, Catherine. 2007. *Dispatches From the Color Line: The Press and Multiracial America.* Albany, NY: State University of New York Press.

Twine, France Winddance and Jonathan Warren. (eds). 2000. *Racing Research, Researching Race: Methodological Dilemmas in Critical Race Studies.* New York: NYU Press.

Valentine, Gill. 2002. "People Like Us: Negotiating Sameness and Difference in the Research Process" in Pamela Moss (ed.). *Feminist Geography in Practice: Research and Methods.* London: Blackwell, 116–27.

12 Situating mixed race politics

Suki Ali

Introduction

In 2001, the UK introduced the 'Mixed' category to the Census. This move came as a result of consultation with some user groups, and a recognition of the limits of the existing 'monoracial' or 'monoethnic' categories which had to that point left individuals who claimed some kind of multiple heritage with no option but to tick the box 'Other'. The resulting data show the young age of this group, and indicate that it is one of the fastest growing 'ethnic groups' in the UK. The statistics have generated a great deal of attention within the national context. Interested parties include academics and activists, policy makers and practitioners working in fields such as social care, education, criminal justice and health provision to name but a few. Alongside academic interest in the theoretical and empirical particularities of mixedness and mixing, there have been numerous groups and individuals keen to put mixed race issues and experiences onto the UK's racial map. While the US has for many years been debating the potentials and pitfalls of a 'multiracial' or 'mixed race' movement, the term 'movement' has not taken off in the UK.[1] This chapter will briefly explore the developments of mixed race politics in the US and contrast these with the UK. It will ask what a 'mixed race politics' might be, what purpose might it serve, and who it might involve. Such questions inevitably invoke further questions about group and individual identities, modes of affiliation, collective and individual struggles for recognition, and rights to (self) representation. I argue that rather than beginning by assuming that there can and should be a singular form of mixed race politics, we need to be more concerned about the wider, situated politics of mixedness. The most important aspect to these politics should be an awareness of the ongoing problems of racialisation and cultural and ethnic absolutism which are contested within complex social relations of unequal and discriminatory differentiation in any given site. Although the chapter uses the US and UK as examples, it is arguing for a non-site specific set of principles that inform a contingent approach to mixed race politics as a reflexive process of engagement with these issues. Such an approach allows for transnational dialogues rather than the uncritical importation of extra-national thinking.

Race mixing and communities of mixedness

The histories of race and race mixing that have impacted upon the current (mixed) race politics in the US and UK have both similarities and distinctions that need to be considered when thinking about their contemporary mixed race politics. In the US, W.E.B. DuBois suggested that 'The problem of the twentieth century is the problem of the color line' (1995 [1903]: 41). While these words are of course powerful and in many ways prescient they are most pertinent to particular understandings of race and community in which 'lines' are drawn and re-drawn in a public, political sphere. Despite a global sensibility and a reference to gradations of racial schema, as an African-American writing in the US in 1903, the 'color' issue for DuBois and his contemporaries was often more immediately focused upon struggles between white and black. The discussions of the 'racial formations' of the nation have been dominated by the history of slavery and segregation and the near genocide of the Native American peoples (Omi and Winant 1986; Todorov 1992; Goldberg 2002; Smith 2005; Hoxie 2008). As a former British colony, the foundation of the modern US state has been central in structuring the politics of race in the US through formal segregation in all social spheres, and a legal prohibition on inter-racial marriage. Political resistance to slavery, oppression and disenfranchisement has been both highly organised and collectivised. The new social movements of the 1960s including the civil rights and Black Power movements became instrumental in the changes to the rights and responsibilities of minority groups in the US. The US constitution resulted in the development of complex national, ethnic and racial formations taking diverse geographic, socio-cultural and political forms. The US has a longer established history of national and ethnic 'hyphenated' identities such as African American, and whiteness has been an unstable category. For example, Polish, Italian and Irish Americans have become white through a process of social and economic assimilation (often at the expense of other racialised minorities; see Roediger 1990, 1994), whereas Asian Americans were first considered 'white' and then 'de-naturalised' (Chan 2003).

In the UK the 'line' was never drawn as clearly or precisely as in the US, primarily because it was not indelibly marked upon the social fabric by legislation. Being indefinite it thus provided the space itself from which to contend 'race'. Michael Banton suggests that it is more appropriate to speak of a 'colour scale' in Britain where individuals were not only ranked by 'colour' but also by socio-economic status (Banton 2008: 42). Inter-marriage and race mixing have been recorded in Britain since at least the 1500s (see e.g. Tizard and Phoenix 1993; Alibhai-Brown and Montagu 1992; Olumide 2002; Caballero in this volume), and in 1614 in the US. However, the US state of Virginia enacted the first law prohibiting inter-racial marriage in 1662 (Zack 1993: 78). In the latter part of the twentieth century, Britain's complex colonial and imperial history continued to impact upon migration and settlement, dominating immigration policy and race relations. Post World War II many people were recruited from the former colonies to fill shortfalls in labour (Solomos 2003). The last two decades of the twentieth century also saw an intensification in 'globalising processes' which further increased 'flows' of people, politics and capital across national borders.

It might seem inevitable that with increasing racial and ethnic diversity in both the US and the UK more people would claim mixed heritage or identity. Whatever the reasons, there are now significant numbers of people claiming labels such as 'mixed race', and setting up organisations that deal with issues around mixed race identity formation, but also often aiming to develop a sense of 'community' and solidarity amongst mixed race people. These sentiments undoubtedly arise in part from the lack of social, cultural and linguistic resources for thinking about mixedness many people have experienced as part of their formative years. As a child growing up in the 1960s and 1970s, I experienced very little if any discussion of mixedness in either social or educational settings. Likewise, as a student in the late 1980s and early 1990s, mixed race was simply not on the 'racial agenda'. In the 1980s, political solidarities were mostly based upon 'monoracial' positions and collectivising under the political category 'Black' was seen as the best way to challenge racism (Back and Solomos 2000). Talking about mixedness was seen to undermine anti-racist struggle, and to enable a racial privilege that pushed those who could 'pass' as white up the social ladder, which meant simultaneously pushing those who were black and brown back down it. Through this period the politics of solidarity shifted and the category of 'Black' fragmented. Categories emerged such as Afro/African-Caribbean, and latterly Black British, British Asian (which include the wide variety of ethnic, cultural and national groups from South Asia) and British-born Chinese to name but three. Today the concept of multiplicity encompasses 'race', culture and religion, and contemporary forms of racism and xenophobia which now often engage with 'Islamophobia' and hostility to 'new migrants' from Eastern Europe (Alexander 2002). However, it is clear that the common thread of these histories is now woven into the fabric of racialised societies which are dominated by the possibilities and failures of multiculturalism. In the US these debates have been intensified by the election of Barack Obama as the first black president (see below). In the UK, they are focused on issues of community cohesion, citizenship and national identity, 'home-grown terror' and the need to manage what is referred to as 'hyper-diversity'. These questions of community building and nation building as they relate to mixedness are explored further below.

The development of a mixed race movement is tied into the idea of a mixed race community. In the US the multiracial movement has been subject to intense scrutiny with scholars and activists debating the relative merits and disadvantages to such a collective approach. Academics have focused both on the challenges to theories of race that multiraciality offers, as well as on the ways in which multiracial identities need to be understood as distinct from those of monoracial identities (Ifekwunigwe 2004; Zack 1993; Root 1996;

Dalmage 2004). Some see multiraciality as an opportunity to deconstruct and dismantle ideologies of race (Root 1992: 10–11). Others caution that 'to see mixture and hybridisation as inherently opposed to racial absolutism and essentialism is quite wrong' (Wade 2004: 356). I would also argue that similar kinds of analyses used to understand so-called multiraciality can and should be bought to bear on so-called monoracial positions. However, this makes thinking about community and its politics a complex area with which to engage.

The political impetus behind the move to gain recognition for mixed race individuals may not strictly fulfil some academic definitions of a 'movement' per se, but it is a term used in a more quotidian fashion. Jon Spencer (1997) looked at the development of the groups that were politically active campaigning during the 1990s for the recognition of mixedness in the US Census of 2000. He argued that 'Political activism is the major factor that distinguishes the contemporary multiracialist groups from the groups that existed in the earlier part of the [twentieth] century' (Spencer 1997: 20). He compared the multiracial movement in the US to the developments leading to the institution of the 'Coloured' category in South Africa. Not surprisingly, given the different histories of the two countries, his basis for comparison was criticised, but his assertion about political engagement being a key shift was perhaps valid. Many of the groups that had campaigned for change were only loosely connected, if at all, and might better be described as interest groups. The members of groups who argued for self-definition that incorporated complex affiliations often expressed these in quite personalised ways, at a micro-level. Objections to multiracialists have included several arguments including those suggesting racial purity is illogical and so African Americans have always been mixed and therefore to claim increases in numbers or a biracial baby boom are erroneous (Spencer 2004); that the 'mark one or more' move would make ethnic monitoring impossible and thus further disadvantage already disadvantaged groups (Small 2001; Spickard 1992); and that the basis of the movement is individualistic (Thompson 2011; DaCosta 2007). It has also been argued that the movement continues to hold problematic alliances with conservative 'colour-blind' politics. Thus in a review of Heather Dalmage's (2004) edited collection on multiraciality in the US after the 2000 Census changes, Wilma Peebles-Wilkins asserts that:

> The multiracial movement is comprised of mixed race families who attempt to promote social justice through organised political and other activities which de-emphasises race. … the movement's ultimate goal is to alter racial thinking in this country [USA] and to *promote color blind world views.*
>
> (Peebles-Wilkins 2006: 263 emphasis added)

This kind of critique seeks to defend a civil rights agenda by arguing that the movement, in effect, suggests that we should not think about race. It points to tensions in the disparate coalitions that formed part of the movement, and how they also reflect disparate academic perspectives on race and ethnicity. It mixes an idea that race is not a simple scientific fact, with a desire to engage with the politics of race. It argues that to hope for a race-free future, is to argue for 'colour blindness' as if 'colour' and 'race' were equivalent and the strategy for eliminating the one is to refuse to 'see' the other. Clearly for those who are struggling to deconstruct ideas of race in all the multitude of ways in which they are thought, practised and lived, this is perhaps a misreading of the theory, and a hijacking of a committed anti-racist politics.

Another issue that is evident here is a privileging of black/white politics, yet the US Census also revealed 'dramatic growth of and increasing visibility of Hispanics and Asians' (Omi 2001: 245). The rise in Asian and Asian-mixed identities are more complex than they appear at first glance. Asian in the US means those of Far East Asian, South Asian and Pacific Islander origins, and there are increasing numbers of people claiming 'hapa' as an identity. Although originally a term that meant a mix of indigenous Hawaiian and white, the term now incorporates multiple mixed-Asian identities (Williams-León and Nakashima 2001). Hispanics/Latinos are also identified in 'race' categories as well, making this a particularly interesting group (Alcoff 2006; Bonilla-Silva 2002, 2009; Golash-Boza and Darity 2008).[2] Despite the idea that many Hispanic identities, such as Mexican, are fundamentally mixed, nearly half chose to identify racially as 'white' and only 2 per cent claimed black, which it has been argued shows evidence of the expansion of and continued desirability of whiteness (Gallagher 2004; Holloway *et al.* in this volume). We should be cautious as ever about the use of statistics, as they tell us nothing about how or why respondents identify in such ways (Song and Hashem 2010), or whether they stay with these identifications, but such changes in formal responses and their interpretations are interesting in and of themselves. Another area of particularity in the US debates is that of the position of Native Americans and the issue of blood quantum. Sturm has argued that 'the legitimacy of racially hybrid Native Americans is questioned more than that of other ethnic groups' and that the requirement of proof of belonging through blood is special treatment that 'acknowledges the federal government's unique relationship with Native American nations as semi-sovereign entities' (Sturm 2002: 3, 8). This is a complex area which raises important questions for the black/white framing of racial politics in the US.

Some argue that the 2000 US Census data and changing political climate show the expansion of a mid-range acceptable group of 'honorary whites', indicating a coming tri-racial system in US race politics (Bonilla-Silva 2004). But African Americans and other black people from Africa and the Caribbean are more clearly demarcated as black, and continue to disproportionately occupy the lower rungs of socio-economic achievement. Whiteness is still a privilege which results in socio-economic benefits (Hunter 2005) so it seems the polarising nature of the black/white system can still incorporate the emerging complexity of racial identifications.

Some of this difficult racial politics was evident in discussions about Barack Obama's campaign for the US presidency and his subsequent election. US social commentator Deborah Dickerson (2007) wrote a scathing article entitled 'Colorblind: Why Obama is not Black'. In it she critiques Obama's pale-skinned appearance, his white mother, absent Muslim father and privileged childhood lived in part outside the US. In her view Obama's mixedness is a further social privilege. For her, Obama steps into the benefits that have been borne out of black struggle through the civil rights movement without having paid his dues, thus he cannot ever be black in her terms. His own claim to blackness is 'inauthentic' and a sop to white liberal guilt. Certainly, the election of Obama, leading to the much-touted idea of the US as 'postracial', could be seen as wishful thinking or a deliberate refusal to engage the ongoing racial inequalities and racism that abound. As Bonilla-Silva states 'Obama's blackness is becoming whites' new weapon of choice for singing their color-blind lullaby' (Bonilla-Silva 2009: 1076).

We can see similar issues at stake in the UK. Identity has been at the heart of the establishment of many activist groups such as People in Harmony, Intermix and The Inheritance Project. Using the language of rights, and drawing on experience, many of the people involved in these groups claim the right to self-identify. Despite their avowed concerns with the positive nature of this challenge to existing terminologies, they might be termed 'defensive' or 'oppositional' identities, as the right to claim 'mixed race' as an identity stands in opposition to a required tick box that names one 'black', 'Asian' or 'other'. They can also be seen as defensive insofar as they are often perceived as providing positive responses to attacks on family, history, heritage which can potentially cause damage to health and well-being. An example of this work in action comes from the Multiple Heritage Project (MHP) founded in Manchester in 2006. MHP worked with young people to allow them safe spaces in which to talk about their own positions as mixed. Such projects are invaluable in a contemporary climate in which multiculturalism is being presented as entrenching and (re)establishing colour and culture lines. Young people were given the opportunity to explore the meanings that are attached to identity choices and use biographical data to inform and theorise their own lives, drawing on personal and social discourses of race. Their preferred terminology was 'mix'd' – something which alludes to the artistic and creative potentials of self-production and representation, and they are now using this collective name and continue to explore these issues with parents, educators and other agency professionals.

It might be helpful to think about the rise in collective mixed race identities in the UK as a shift in the 'social imaginary' (Appadurai 1996). One aspect of this is to challenge the idea that mixed identities are somehow inauthentic, another celebrates people who have some kind of mixed heritage. This too is problematic, as the exoticisation and objectification of certain types of mixedness continues apace. Some of this may come from the mixed race movement itself. As Spencer (1997) and others have noted in the US, many 'monoracial' whites were key activists in the development of the mixed race movement, and this requires careful scrutiny of issues of inter-racial, -ethnic and -cultural sociality and kinship. Anger has been expressed that many claims to mixedness, often made by white parents, are not based upon white supremacy but of mixed 'superiority'; smarter, cleverer and – most often – more beautiful than monoracial people (Spencer 1997, 2004). In addition, it is claimed that the collectivisation of these beautiful people is the 'future of race' and that this is a good thing (Ali 2005). Two people who claim different racialised identities, in a partnership they consider to be familial, with or without children, can of course describe this as a mixed race family. However, I would suggest that in societies that 'see race' as important, there may be differences in how 'monoracial' people in inter-racial relationships experience mixing and how those who are required to negotiate such multiplicity within a singular embodied self experience this. There are no simple ways to think about the impact of these issues. For me they are part of the ongoing reflexivity required of all of us who live in racialising societies which are still plagued by racism and prejudice.

Recognising mixed race

It is clear that recognition of mixedness as a lived category of experience is framed within complex and contradictory elements that lie at the heart of discussions about the making and shaping of racial and ethnic groups. Further, in the US and the UK during the twentieth century, the political recognition of mixedness has become a key issue. Charles Taylor's analysis of multiculturalism and the politics of recognition may be pertinent here. Taylor argues that a classical liberal model of authenticity requires individuals to be true to themselves, and that this *true* identity is crucial for self-actualisation. However, he argues that identities are dialogic, formed in relation between self and society, and in order to be fulfilled, the self must be recognised by others. Building on the work of feminists and postcolonialists he suggests that non-recognition and mis-recognition are forms of harm, or even oppression (Taylor 1992). But for Taylor the politics of recognition has two elements: (1) the politics of universalism which comes from the recognition of equal dignity of all humans and (2) the rise of the politics of difference. Under the first, all citizens have the right to be recognised, and most importantly, this recognition is central to the achievement of equality and social justice. For the second, the recognition of difference might be essential in order to achieve equality, and is not unconnected to the first. In both we see a need to address universal rights in relation to particular identities. Taylor is most interested in group rights, specifically minority ethnic and cultural group rights. He discusses 'rights' in their broadest terms, and considers equality in relation to a wide range of social provisions and outcomes in areas such as poverty, education and health.

Taylor's work has, of course, both merits and limitations. He uses a particular model of a rational, individualistic citizen, and his account of communities or groups (particularly those based upon some kind of cultural identification) can appear to be somewhat ossified. However, a dialogic perspective reveals how the right to name oneself 'mixed race' or 'of mixed heritage' raises the blurring of boundaries between public and private spheres. It is not enough to be able to narrate a 'private' tale of genealogy or kinship, such a position must be acknowledged in the public sphere. In the US, this leads to difficult debates about racial categorisation and anti-racism. In the UK, the importance of the political takes a slightly different form. The inclusion of 'the mixed category' can be seen as a victory in terms of recognition. However it has raised further questions in relation to the issue of the collectivisation and representation of mixedness. For example, 'the mixed category' in all its heterogeneity has become a group. In a 2006 speech, the then head of the Commission for Equalities and Human Rights, Trevor Phillips, cited the speed of demographic change in the UK as one of the major barriers to a workable multiculturalism. In his talk he noted the 'astonishing rise in the numbers of mixed race Britons' who will become 'the single largest minority group in the country' (Phillips 2006). Phillips cannot be said to speak for mixed race Britons, but his talk and his interpretation of the Census information points to the paradoxical effects of recognition. He invokes the notion of a singular minority ethnic group named 'mixed'. Whether or not we might consider this problematic, he felt it is important because what he called mixed race Britons are an unusual group in that they are both particularly successful, but also particularly at risk. In support of his argument, research in the UK shows 'the mixed-race population' are more likely to be underachieving at school (Tikly *et al.* 2004), children are disproportionately represented in the care system (Barn 2007) and in the prison system (Reza and Magill 2006) as well as being at greater risk of crime than all other ethnic groups (Salisbury and Upson 2004), yet are achieving in other areas of education and employment (Platt in this volume). And finally, Phillips suggests the problem for many mixed race Britons is one of 'identity stripping', not a common phrase, but one that is as evocative as his pronouncement that these individuals are at risk of finding themselves 'marooned between communities' (Phillips 2006).

While we should not read Phillips' comments as representative of anything other than his own position, and it is certainly open to contestation, it raises some interesting points. Firstly, we should perhaps be concerned that the incredible heterogeneity of individuals who responded to the Census are here collectivised into a singular minority ethnic group when work in the UK has consistently pointed to the ways in which mixed race identities are experienced as varied and diverse, and are, as with all identities, simultaneously produced through and with a range of other kinds of social differentiation (Song 2010; Bradford 2006). Secondly, the continued tendency to either idealise or pathologise mixed people is evident in the discussion of achievement in employment and of problematic family forms. Better or worse than others, but not simply equivalent – mixed race becomes a marker of difference. And finally, the comments about identity echo much older concerns about the potential psychic damage to mixed individuals their multiplicity may confer upon them – a form of identificatory outsiderness which has been undermined by empirical research.[3] My reading of his comments is that the important shift in his rhetoric is that rather than an inside/out model of some kind of inherent psychosis, Phillips alludes to the formative power of racial and ethnic communities. His account suggests that mixed race people are banished from existing communities and thus have no community. In his formulation, recognition as mixed at the public, macro-level of Census data has done nothing to alleviate the problems at the meso- and micro-levels. At these levels, it is precisely the desire for mixedness that is problematic, and is a potential barrier to inclusion in existing communities. Following the logic of this argument, we might conclude that under such conditions it would hardly be surprising that mixed race people would want to form their own communities. The problems that face many mixed race people are exacerbated by ideas of race that result in 'communities' defining themselves in such exclusive and purist terms (see McKenzie in this volume). Phillips seems to elide race and ethnicity, and maps them on to cultural communities – what does this mean for an individual who is raised with ethnic, cultural and racial plurality?

As Anthias and Yuval-Davis (1993) have suggested, in its broadest terms, belonging to ethnic collectivities requires one to be able to muster the appropriate resources in order to be a member of the group. In the case of many mixed race people, despite being able to do that, they may still be seen as inauthentic in some way. This indicates an ongoing question about the ways in which all these aspects – race, ethnicity and culture – of identity are invoked such that they continue to assume some kind of prior, given 'pure' or 'singular' or certainly definable and bounded 'thing'. Quite simply, both those in favour of, for example, simple understandings of 'the Chinese community' and those who argue for the possibilities for solidarity within 'the mixed race community' are in danger of investing in the 'myths of origins', whether or not they are seeking to evade charges of ethnic absolutism. The price of recognition might also be a form of representation that is either a glorification or pathologisation of mixedness. One newer group, Turquoise, had this statement on its web-pages:

> What we do and Why we do it:
>
> We are a group of young adults with a mixed heritage. We are taking a leading role in promoting mixed heritage within Britain. We recognise that there is a growing population of mixed individuals in Britain, and are keen to promote our own experiences born from embracing, celebrating and identifying with our multiple heritages. Our vision is to engage with and promote the mixed heritage community so we can celebrate who we are by being able to identify with and see the achievements of mixed people in UK society. We are establishing a structured

> mechanism for mixed heritage people to come together to network, share their experiences, ideas, and have debates and discussions about their achievements.
>
> (Turquoise Association, n.d.)

This group of largely professional young adults seek to inspire a new generation of mixed individuals. They are concerned with including everyone in this group under the heading of community, and under their list of activities request global ambassadors and entrepreneurs. There is a point under their ethical statement at which they note that some vulnerable people suffer discrimination over race, gender or disability and that this is unacceptable. Clearly the members feel strongly about the need for group recognition, and representation in many different forms. But where is the explicit anti-racist sentiment in this statement? How might we feel about the idea of 'promoting' mixed race people? In spite of evident good intentions, such a remit might be considered by some the result of a neo-liberal, individualistic, anti-racist sentiment that fails to fully engage the structured forms of inequality that face *all* minority ethnic groups in the UK, and illustrates concerns about the racial politics behind this as outlined above (see also Mahtani in this volume). While sympathising with the group's ideal of recognition and self-representation, the form it takes here could be interpreted as apolitical, and veering towards the 'celebratory' at the expense of critical engagement with the diverse representations and experiences of mixedness (particularly classed, geographically contingent, and hetero/gendered), and most importantly, the processes of racialisation that form them.

Conclusions: towards a situated politics of mixedness?

The distinct development of forms and processes of racialisation in the US and the UK have led to different kinds of political struggle for recognition for those who name themselves in the different sites as variously multiracial, mixed race, biracial, having multiple heritage and so on. The struggles over the names also point to the different histories of race making, and it would seem misguided to attempt to transport models from one site to another. It is more important to consider the extremely complex and contingent discursive sites and practices that produce 'race' and 'mixed race' in their many forms. Specificity does not mean that we might not see points of similarity and patterns of congruence, but the need to understand the particulars of what forms racialised hierarchies is what matters most to the project of dismantling them. We might better engage understandings of mixed race by situating them within theoretical frameworks that are engaged with understanding the wider politics of belonging in multiracial, multiethnic and multicultural societies. The border crossings that are inherent to a discussion of mixed race require a political engagement with the ways in which mixing is managed and mixedness produced within sites which consist of multiple time-lines for indigenous, migrant and settler populations.

The mixed race movement in the US was explicitly engaged with a politics of recognition, which called for changes to the Census to allow more flexible and inclusive social identities – with limited success. In the UK discussions took place in a less organised political fashion, and also resulted in recognition in the Census – again not to the satisfaction of all involved (Aspinall 2003, 2009). The context for these inclusions are described by social commentators as periods of rapid change, and concerns about the ways in which racial and ethnic relations are managed in multicultural societies. Fears which have been expressed in the US about the collectivisation of mixed race echo wider concerns about the ways in which identity-based movements may weaken the possibilities of coalition politics. Although the UK has not seen the same kind of organised claim to recognition, it can also be seen to be guided by similar concerns to the right of self-identification as the basis for a form of self-actualisation. However, as Linda Alcoff says of the US context, 'Strongly felt identities *in reality* do not uniformly lead to the political disasters the critics portend because identities *in reality* are not what the critics understand them to be' (Alcoff 2006: 41), and identity-based interest groups need not inevitably lead to separatism in US race politics. It is the fear of separatism of various groups that underpins the discussions about community formation and multiculturalism in the UK. Yet, I would argue that the mixed race population (if one can call it that), while developing networks and collective forms of identification, does not currently perceive itself as a community per se. The most important thing is that even if mixed race people do perceive themselves as a community, this does not inevitably mean that this community will be 'separate' from other issue-based groups or more importantly from other minority groups organising on the basis of race, ethnicity and/or culture. What is more of an issue is the position of mixedness vis-à-vis hierarchical organisations of social differentiation. An understanding of the hierarchical nature of social organisation needs to underpin a politics of mixing, and this in turn should inform what I am calling a situated politics of mixedness. A situated politics of mixedness recognises that all knowledge is partial and situated (Haraway 1991); the need to consider the 'politics of location' (Frankenberg and Mani 1993; Kaplan 1994); and builds upon a 'situated politics of belonging' (Yuval-Davis *et al.* 2006).

Considering a situated politics of mixedness requires us to pay close attention not only to the complexities of contemporary positionalities, but how such positionalities have arisen. In the examples I have drawn upon, the US and the UK, the histories are in some ways intertwined, especially through colonialism and imperialism, yet they are distinct and specific to the social conditions of advantage and disadvantage that attend them. Forms of alignment and refusal, whether named as racial, or ethnic, or cultural, require an analysis of power and privilege, and a critical engagement with the politics of recognition. I would argue that there is clearly nothing intrinsically problematic about collectivising as mixed race, indeed individuals finding solidarity with others, rather than being defined as 'other', may be crucial for one's sense of self. However, it is as important to recognise the power dynamics at play in which kinds of identification are opened up and which are foreclosed in this process, how these are intercut by other kinds of inequality, and whether these processes feed into the perpetuation of racial hierarchies within societies. This is as true of mixed identities and politics as it is of any other. Recognition is not necessarily a problematic goal, but I do not believe it should be an end in itself, nor should it be achieved at the expense of a continued engagement with the wider politics of race and racism within any given site.

Notes

1 Questions of terminology have been discussed extensively elsewhere. The variability in terminologies is not only national, but regional and local. In addition, there has been discussion about the discrepancies between 'official' and 'academic' terminologies and those used in everyday situations, with the preferred term remaining 'mixed race' in the UK as opposed to terms like 'multiracial' and 'biracial' in the US (see e.g. Tizard and Phoenix 1993; Ifekwunigwe 1999; Parker and Song 2001; Ali 2003; Edwards and Caballero 2008; Caballero 2010; McKenzie in this volume).

2 There is debate and dissent about the use of the terms 'Hispanic' and 'Latino/a' and I use the differing versions in accordance with the materials in which they arise.

3 This has been a key feature of concerns about mixed race identities and is discussed in the UK context in Tizard and Phoenix 1993; Ali 2003; Ifekwunigwe 1999; Parker and Song 2001; Alibhai-Brown 2001; Song and Aspinall in this volume; and in relation to families in, for example Olumide 2002; Caballero *et al.* 2008; Edwards *et al.* 2010. In the US, for example, Root 1992; Root 1996; Ifekwunigwe 2004; Rockquemore and Brunsma 2002.

References

Alcoff, L. (2006) *Visible Identities: Race, Gender and the Self*, Oxford: Oxford University Press.

Alexander, C. (2002): 'Beyond Black: Rethinking the Colour/Culture Divide', *Ethnic and Racial Studies*, 25 (4): 552–71.

Ali, S. (2003) *Mixed-Race, Post-Race: Gender, New Ethnicities and Cultural Practices*, Oxford: Berg.

——(2005) 'Uses of the Exotic: Body, Narrative, Mixedness' in Alexander, C. and Knowles, C. (eds) *Making Race Matter: Bodies, Space and Identity*, Basingstoke: Palgrave Macmillan.

Alibhai-Brown, Y. (2001) *Mixed Feelings: The Complex Lives of Mixed Race Britons*, London: The Women's Press.

Alibhai-Brown, Y. and Montagu, A. (1992) *The Colour of Love: Mixed Race Relationships*, London: Virago.

Anthias, F. and Yuval-Davis, N. (1993) *Racialized Boundaries: Race, Nation, Gender, Colour and Class, and the Anti-Racist Struggle*, London: Routledge.

Appadurai, A. (1996) *Modernity at Large: Cultural Dimensions of Globalisation*, Minneapolis, MN: University of Minnesota Press.

Aspinall, P. (2003) 'The Conceptualisation and Categorisation of Mixed Race/Ethnicity in Britain and North America: Identity Options and the Role of the State', *International Journal of Intercultural Relations*, 27: 269–96.

——(2009) '"Mixed Race", "Mixed Origins" or What?', *Anthropology Today*, 25 (2): 3–8.

Back, L. and Solomos, J. (eds) (2000) *Theories of Race and Racism*, London and New York: Routledge.

Banton, M. (2008) 'Problem-Finding in Ethnic and Racial Studies' in Eade, J., Barrett, M., Floud, C. and Race, R. (eds) *Advancing Multiculturalism, Post 7/7*, Newcastle: Cambridge Scholars.

Barn, R. (2007) '"Race", Ethnicity and Child Welfare: A Fine Balancing Act', *British Journal of Social Work*, 37 (8): 1425–34.

Bonilla-Silva, E. (ed.) (2002) 'The Latin Americanization of US Race Relations', *Special Issue of Race and Society*, 5 (1): 1–114.

——(2004) 'From Bi-Racial to Tri-Racial: Towards a New System of Racial Stratification in the USA', *Ethnic and Racial Studies,* 27 (6): 931–950.

——(2009) 'Are the Americas "Sick with Racism" or Is It a Problem at the Poles? A Reply to Christina A. Sue', *Ethnic and Racial Studies*, 32 (6): 1071–82.

Bradford, B. (2006) *Who Are the "Mixed" Ethnic Group?* London: Office for National Statistics.

Brown, M.K. (2003) *Whitewashing Race: The Myth of a Color-Blind Society*, George Gund Foundation Book in African American Studies, Berkeley, CA: University of California Press.

Caballero, C. (2010) *Lone Mothers of Children From Mixed Racial And Ethnic Backgrounds: A Case Study*, Bristol: Single Parent Action Network Publications.

Caballero, C., Edwards, R. and Puthussery, S. (2008) *Parenting 'Mixed' Children: Negotiating Difference and Belonging in Mixed Race, Ethnicity and Faith Families*, York: York Publishing Services Ltd, Joseph Rowntree Foundation.

Chan, S. (2003) *Remapping Asian American History*, Lanham, MD: AltaMira Press.

DaCosta, K. (2007) *Making Multiracials: State, Family, and Market in the Redrawing of the Color Line*, Stanford, CA: Stanford University Press.

Dalmage, H. (ed.) (2004) *The Politics of Multiracialism: Challenging Racial Thinking*, Albany, NY: State University of New York Press.

Dickerson, D. (2007) 'Colorblind: Why Obama is not Black', *Salon,* http://www.salon.com/opinion/feature/2007/01/22/obama/ (accessed 17.9.09).

DuBois, W.E.B. (1995 [1903]) *The Souls of Black Folk*, New York: Signet Books.

Edwards, R. and Caballero, C. (2008) 'What's in a Name? An Exploration of the Significance of Personal Naming of "Mixed" Children for Parents from Different Racial, Ethnic and Faith Backgrounds', *The Sociological Review*, 56 (1): 39–60.

Edwards, R., Caballero, C. and Puthussery, S. (2010) 'Parenting Children from "Mixed" Racial, Ethnic and Faith Backgrounds: Typifications of Difference and Belonging', *Ethnic and Racial Studies*, 33 (6): 949–67.

Frankenberg, R. and Mani, L. (1993) 'Crosscurrents, Cross Talk: Race, "Postcoloniality" and the Politics of Location', *Cultural Studies*, 7(2): 292–310.

Gallagher, C.A. (2004) 'Racial Redistricting: Expanding the Boundaries of Whiteness' in Dalmage, H. (ed.) *The Politics of Multiracialism: Challenging Racial Thinking*, Albany, NY: State University of New York Press.

Golash-Boza, T. and Darity Jr, W. (2008) 'Latino Racial Choices: The Effects of Skin Colour and Discrimination on Latinos' and Latinas' Racial Self-Identifications', *Ethnic and Racial Studies,* 31 (5): 899–934.

Goldberg, D. (2002) *The Racial State*, Oxford: Blackwell.

Haraway, D. (1991) 'Situated Knowledges: The Science Question in Feminism and The Privilege of the Partial Perspective' in Haraway, D. (ed.) *Simians, Cyborgs and Women: The Reinvention of Nature,* New York: Routledge.

Hoxie, F.E. (2008) 'Retrieving the Red Continent: Settler Colonialism and the History of American Indians in the US', *Ethnic and Racial Studies,* 31 (6): 1153–67.

Hunter, M.L (2005) *Race, Gender and the Politics of Skin Tone*, New York: Routledge.

Ifekwunigwe, J.O. (1999) *Scattered Belongings: The Cultural Paradoxes of 'Race', Nation and Gender*, London and New York: Routledge.

——(2004) *Mixed Race Studies: A Reader*, London and New York: Routledge.

Kaplan, C. (1994) 'The Politics of Location as Transnational Feminist Critical Practice' in Grewal, I. and Kaplan, C. (eds) *Scattered Hegemonies: Postmodernity and Transnational Feminist Practices*, Minneapolis, MN: University of Minnesota Press.

Olumide, J. (2002) *Raiding the Gene Pool: The Social Construction of Mixed Race*, London: Pluto Press.

Omi, M.A. (2001) 'The Changing Meaning of Race' in Smelser, N.I., Wilson, W.J. and Mitchell, J. (eds) *America Becoming: Racial Trends and their Consequences Volume 1*, Washington, DC: National Academic Press.

Omi, M. and Winant, H. (1986) *Racial Formation in the United States: From the 1960s to the 1980s*, London and New York: Routledge.

Parker, D. and Song, M. (eds) (2001) *Rethinking 'Mixed Race'*, London: Pluto Press.

Peebles-Wilkins, W. (2006) 'Review of Heather Dalmage (ed.) (2004) *The Multiracial Movement*', *Journal of Sociology and Social Welfare,* 33 (1): 262–64.

Phillips, T. (2006) 'The state of the nation's race relations'. Speech delivered at Commission for Racial Equality RACE CONVENTION 2006. Partial transcript available at http://79.170.40.182/billgreenshields.org.uk/index.php?option=com_content&view=article&id=58:cre-race-convention-qsleepwalking-to-segregation-or-strength-through-diversityq&catid=14:national-campaigns&Itemid=29 (accessed 14.1.12).

Reza, B. and Magill, C. (2006) *Race and the Criminal Justice System: An Overview of the Complete Statistics*, London: Home Office Publications.

Rockquemore, K.A. and Brunsma, D.L. (2002) *Beyond Black: Biracial Identity in America*, Thousand Oaks, CA: Sage.

Roediger, D. (1990) *The Wages of Whiteness: Race and the Making of the American Working Class*, London: Verso.

——(1994) *The Abolition of Whiteness: Essays on Race, Politics and Working Class History*, London: Verso.

Root, M.P.P. (ed.) (1992) *Racially Mixed People in America*, New York: Sage.

——(1996) *The Multiracial Experience: Racial Borders as the New Frontier*, New York: Sage.

Salisbury, H. and Upson, A. (2004) *Ethnicity, Victimisation and Worry about Crime: Findings from the 2001/02 and 2002/03 British Crime Surveys*, London: Home Office Publications.

Small, S. (2001) 'Interrogating the Mixed Race Movement in the USA' in Parker, D. and Song, M. (eds) *Rethinking 'Mixed Race'*, London: Pluto Press.

Smith, A. (2005) *Conquest: Sexual Violence and American Indian Genocide*, Cambridge, MA: Southend Press.

Solomos, J. (2003) *Race and Racism in Britain*, Basingstoke: Palgrave.

Song, M. (2010) 'Is There a Mixed Race Group in Britain? The Diversity of Multiracial Identification and Experience', *Critical Social Policy*, 30 (3): 337–58.

Song, M. and Hashem, F. (2010) 'What Does "White" Mean? Interpreting the Choice of Race by Mixed Race Young People in Britain', *Sociological Perspectives*, 53 (2): 287–92.

Spencer, J.M. (1997) *The New Colored People: The Mixed-Race Movement in America*, New York and London: New York University Press.

Spencer, R. (2004) 'Beyond Pathology and Cheerleading: Insurgency, Dissolution, and Complicity in the Multiracial Idea' in Dalmage, H.M. (ed.) *The Politics of Multiracialism: Challenging Racial Thinking*, New York: SUNY Press.

Spickard, P.R. (1992) 'The Illogic of American Racial Categories' in Root, M.P.P. (ed.) *Racially Mixed People in America*, New York: Sage Publications.

Sturm, C. (2002) *Blood Politics: Race, Culture and Identity in the Cherokee Nation of Oklahoma*, London, Berkeley and LA: University of California Press.

Taylor, C. (1992) *Multiculturalism and the Politics of Recognition*, Princeton, NJ: Princeton University Press.

Thompson, D. (2011) 'Making (Mixed-)Race: Census Politics and the Emergence of Multiracial Multiculturalism in the United States, Great Britain and Canada', *Ethnic and Racial Studies*, 16 (1): 75–94.

Tikly, L., Caballero, C., Haynes, J., and Hill, J. in association with Birmingham Local Education Authority (2004) *Understanding the Educational Needs of Mixed Heritage Pupils*, London: Department for Education and Skills.

Tizard, B. and Phoenix, A. (1993) *Black, White or Mixed-Race: Race and Racism in the Lives of Young People*, New York and London: Routledge.

Todorov, T. (1992) *The Conquest of America*, New York, HarperCollins.

Turquoise Association (n.d.), http://turquoiseassociation.org/index.html (accessed 30.11.09).

Wade, P. (2004) 'Images of Latin American *Mestizaje* and the Politics of Comparison', *Bulletin of Latin American Research*, 23 (3): 355–56.

Williams-León, T. and Nakashima, C. (eds) (2001) *The Sum of Our Parts: Mixed Heritage Asian Americans*, Philadelphia, PA: Temple University Press.

Yuval-Davis, N., Kannabiran, K., and Vietan, U. (eds) (2006) *The Situated Politics of Belonging*, London, New York and New Delhi: Sage.

Zack, N. (1993) *Race and Mixed Race*, Philadelphia, PA: Temple University Press.

Index

Page numbers in *italics* denotes a figure/table